# IMAGING AND URODYNAMICS OF THE LOWER URINARY TRACT

**Uday Patel** MB, ChB, MRCP, FRCR

Consultant Uro-Radiologist
*St George's Hospital and Medical School*
*London, UK*

**David Rickards** FFRDSA, FRCR

Consultant Uro-Radiologist
*University College London Hospitals*
*London, UK*

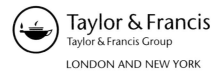
Taylor & Francis
Taylor & Francis Group

LONDON AND NEW YORK

© 2005 Taylor & Francis, an imprint of the Taylor & Francis Group

First published in the United Kingdom in 2005
by Taylor & Francis,
an imprint of the Taylor & Francis Group,
2 Park Square, Milton Park
Abingdon, Oxon OX14 4RN, UK

Tel.:   +44 (0) 20 7017 6000
Fax.:   +44 (0) 20 7017 6699
Website: www.tandf.co.uk

Although every effort has been made to ensure that all owners of copyright material have been
acknowledged in this publication, we would be glad to acknowledge in subsequent reprints or edi-
tions any omissions brought to our attention.

British Library Cataloguing in Publication Data

Data available on application

Library of Congress Cataloging-in-Publication Data

Data available on application

ISBN 1-84184-325-3

Distributed in North and South America by

Taylor & Francis
2000 NW Corporate Blvd
Boca Raton, FL 33431, USA

*Within Continental USA*
Tel.: 800 272 7737; Fax.: 800 374 3401
*Outside Continental USA*
Tel.: 561 994 0555; Fax.: 561 361 6018
E-mail: orders@crcpress.com

Distributed in the rest of the world by
Thomson Publishing Services
Cheriton House
North Way
Andover, Hampshire SP10 5BE, UK
Tel.: +44 (0) 1264 332424
E-mail: salesorder.tandf@thomsonpublishingservices.co.uk

Composition by Parthenon Publishing
Printed and bound by T. G. Hostench S.A., Spain

I

.E

# LOWER URINARY TRACT

# CONTENTS

Preface vii

1. The normal bladder 1

2. Imaging modalities used for assessment of the bladder 7

3. Congenital anomalies of the bladder 25

4. Intraluminal abnormalities of the bladder 29

5. Abnormalities of the bladder wall or mural abnormalities 35

6. Staging of bladder cancer 49

7. Abnormal bladder contour or size 57

8. Functional abnormalities of the bladder 65

9. The normal urethra 87

10. Congenital anomalies of the urethra 97

11. Intraluminal abnormalities and filling defects of the urethra 103

12. Intrinsic abnormalities of the urethral wall 107

13. Lower urinary tract trauma 115

14. Neoplasms of the urethra 123

Bibliography 127
Index 135

# PREFACE

Lower urinary tract symptoms may be the result of a structural or functional abnormality. To consider either in isolation would be an incomplete assessment, but combining anatomical imaging with functional measurement provides a more powerful and complete tool for lower urinary tract investigation. Yet many of the currently available radiological texts concerning lower urinary tract imaging fail to discuss these two aspects in a holistic manner. We hope this book will fill this gap. Although it is written to be as comprehensive as possible, such that it covers the vast majority of lower urinary tract disorders that will be encountered in adult urological practice, it is not meant to replace conventional textbooks of uroradiology. Rather, we have tried to maintain a practical, user-friendly style. Intended for everyday clinical use, it is meant to allow both the trainee and trained radiologist or urologist to plan a logical, yet complete, radiological and dynamic investigation of the lower urinary tract. In this respect it should also be useful for nurse practitioners and other medical staff who commonly manage lower urinary tract disorders.

# 1. THE NORMAL BLADDER

- DEVELOPMENT OF THE BLADDER
- ANATOMY OF THE BLADDER
- PHYSIOLOGY OF THE BLADDER AND MICTURITION

## EMBRYOLOGY OF THE BLADDER

The bladder develops from the urogenital sinus, but the base (or bladder trigone) is of mesonephric duct origin. Development of the bladder commences with the embryonic cloaca or the primitive gut. The cloaca is further subdivided by the urorectal septum, and the anterior division forms the primitive bladder. The mesonephric ducts join the bladder and become the ureters. The upper part of the primitive bladder is continuous with the allantois and urachus, which degenerates into a cord-like structure called the median umbilical ligament. The ligament becomes the urachus. This structure may persist to a variable degree after birth. At birth the bladder is more superior in location than its final position in the adult within the true pelvis.

## ANATOMY OF THE BLADDER (AND PROSTATE)

### The urinary bladder

The urinary bladder has to serve both a storage and periodic expulsive function; its unique neurology and anatomy make it ideally suited for this role.

It lies centrally in the pelvis and although extraperitoneal, the peritoneum reflects over its superior surface (Figure 1.1). When fully distended it is spherical in shape but when partly full it approximates to a more cuboid outline. The bladder base, or trigone, lies inferiorly and is indistinguishable from the rest of the bladder, except that it may be slightly raised, particularly in the male because of the prostate gland. The ureters enter the trigone approximately 2 cm either side of the midline and are identifiable as a slight corrugation on ultrasound imaging as they traverse diagonally through the bladder wall. With full distension, the normal bladder neck may be seen as a slightly open funnel at the base of the bladder. These – the trigone, ureters and bladder neck – are the only fixed landmarks seen on imaging.

The walls of the bladder have been described as having three major components – outer adventitia, intervening detrusor (smooth) muscle and inner

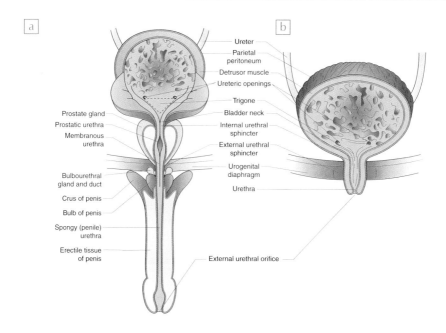

Figure 1.1   The anatomy of the bladder (and also the urethra). (a) Illustrates the anatomy in the male, and (b) that in the female

transitional cell-lined (urothelium) mucous membrane. The detrusor muscles have been described in the past as subdivided into three parts – the outer longitudinal muscle layer, the middle circular muscle and an inner longitudinal layer. However, it has now been proposed that rather than discrete layers as described before, the detrusor muscle is in fact a composite of interlacing muscle fibres following no particular direction. Some of the muscle fibres at the base of the bladder merge with the prostate capsule or the anterior vaginal wall. The urothelium (transitional cell epithelium) lines the inner part of the muscle layer and is continuous with the urothelium of the ureters and urethra.

The interior surface is smooth on full distension, but corrugated when not distended, except around the trigone, which is always smooth because it is a fixed structure. The muscles around the bladder neck fuse to form the internal urethral sphincter, which encircles the upper prostatic urethra (Figure 1.1). In the female the external urethral sphincter lies just below the bladder neck with the uterus posteriorly (the space being the pouch of Douglas or the rectovesical pouch, which often contains a small amount of fluid). In the male the prostate gland lies between the bladder neck and the external urethral sphincter, with the seminal vesicles and rectum as the posterior structures (the rectovesical pouch lies between).

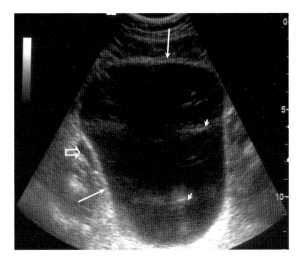

Figure 1.2 An axial ultra-sound view of the bladder and surrounding anatomical structures. The wall of the bladder is indicated by the long arrows. This view was taken with a 3.5-MHz curved array probe. Views of the anterior bladder wall (long vertical arrow) can be improved and internal artefactual shadows (short arrows) can be reduced by the use of harmonic or pulse inversion techniques. The open arrow indicates the right iliac vessels

## Relations of the bladder

Superiorly, the peritoneum separates the bladder from the small and large bowel loops. The anterior surface is extraperitoneal; when empty the retropubic space, with its fat and veins, lies anterior. As the bladder distends the peritoneum is lifted with the superior bladder surface and the anterior abdominal wall, and the rectus sheath with its contents, becomes the anterior relation. Thus, surgically, an extraperitoneal access is possible through an abdominal incision, as long as the organ is well distended. The space of Retzius lies between the anterior bladder wall and the posterior aspect of the pubis symphysis – it is also known as the anterior perivesical space, and is another landmark during pelvic surgery. The inferolateral relations are the obturator nerve and superior vesical vessels, the obturator internus and levator ani muscles (Figure 1.2).

Posterior and inferior relations are gender dependent. In the male the seminal vesicles and the vas deferens separate the bladder from the rectum. A cone of peritoneum lies between the two – the rectovesical pouch – and the inferior relation is the prostate gland. In the female the uterus, the uterine cervix and the vagina lie posteriorly, from superior to inferior. The pouch of Douglas lies between the body of the uterus and the bladder. The most inferior relation is the bladder neck, which leads to the urethra – within the external sphincter and perineal body in the female and within the prostate in the male. The levator ani muscles lie inferolaterally.

## Blood supply of the bladder

The blood supply of the bladder originates from branches of the anterior division of the internal iliac artery. The superior vesical arteries are the dominant supplies but there are further variable and smaller branches arising from the obturator and inferior gluteal arteries, or from the uterine and vaginal arteries in the female. Venous drainage is also variable. The vesical venous plexus drains into the internal iliac, but there are further direct pathways draining into the inferior vena cava, via the ovarian and sacral veins.

## Nerve supply of the bladder

Autonomic fibres from the pelvic plexuses travel with the vessels to the bladder wall. These aspects, as well as further details of the neural control of micturition, are given below.

## The prostate

Some brief details of prostate anatomy are included here because in the male the bladder, particularly functionally, is closely related to this gland. Embryologically, the prostate gland develops from outgrowths of the urogenital sinus and the embryological prostatic urethra.

### Gross anatomy of the prostate

Post-puberty the prostate gland has a volume of up to 25 ml – size being approximately 3.5 cm long or high, 4.0 cm wide and 2.5 cm in anterior to posterior depth – or the size and shape of a walnut. For unknown reasons, though presumably hormones play a role, the gland increases in size and changes shape with age. Like the bladder, the prostate is a retroperitoneal structure, lying anterior to the rectum and inferior to the bladder. Between the gland and the rectum lies Denonvilliers' fascia – an obliterated peritoneal plane. Gland shape conforms to the anatomical limitations of the deep pelvic boundaries and the gland resembles an inverted cone or pyramid. On the sides lie the levator ani and obturator internus muscles. The superior margin, or the base of the gland, lies immediately below the bladder. The most inferior part of the gland is the apex (Figure 1.1), lying just above the urogenital diaphragm, which is a fibrous supporting ring that also contains the urethra and the external urethral sphincter.

The deep pelvis is a restricted space and insufficient to accommodate significant gland enlargement. Beyond a certain size, the gland will preferentially enlarge superiorly, protruding into the bladder base – so-called median lobe enlargement. Enlargement may be substantial and asymmetric and there may be marked distortion of the bladder base and trigone. In the past, the gland was considered as a lobar structure, with right and left lobes, and a midline median lobe. Lobar anatomy is no longer thought to be an accurate representation in the adult, and the gland is now split into three glandular zones – the central, transition and peripheral zones. The neurovascular bundles contain the branch arteries, veins and nerves; and lie posterolaterally.

## Physiology of the bladder and control of micturition

The bladder has a dual physiological role, i.e. storage and expulsion; this requires a complex interaction between the bladder (or the detrusor muscle), the various continence-maintaining muscular sphincters and the urethra. All these actions are under the control of linked neural connections as illustrated in Figure 1.3. Filling

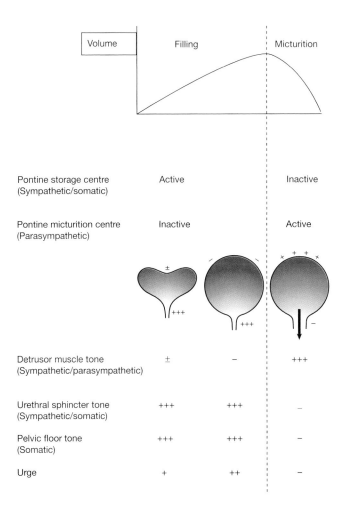

| Volume | Filling | | Micturition |
|---|---|---|---|
| Pontine storage centre (Sympathetic/somatic) | Active | | Inactive |
| Pontine micturition centre (Parasympathetic) | Inactive | | Active |
| Detrusor muscle tone (Sympathetic/parasympathetic) | ± | − | +++ |
| Urethral sphincter tone (Sympathetic/somatic) | +++ | +++ | − |
| Pelvic floor tone (Somatic) | +++ | +++ | − |
| Urge | + | ++ | − |

Figure 1.3   Neural control of bladder storage and expulsion

of the bladder is facilitated by relaxation of the detrusor muscle. Distension on bladder expansion excites low-frequency stimulation of the afferent nerve fibres, and this stimulus is transmitted via the spinal cord to the pontine storage centre. In turn, the pontine storage centre activates the sympathetic and somatic nerve fibres, which facilitate relaxation of the detrusor muscle and contraction of the bladder neck, urethral muscles and the pelvic floor. Thus the bladder fills but is continent.

Increasing bladder expansion further reinforces neural stimuli and sizeable volumes can be stored without urinary leakage. The inherently high bladder compliance means that storage occurs without much increase in intra-bladder pressure, until distension reaches a critical limit, which varies with age or sex, and the afferent nerve fibres fire at a higher frequency. This is conveyed to the higher centres and a desire to micturate reaches higher consciousness. When appropriate, e.g. when in the toilet, the pontine micturition centre takes over from the pontine storage centre. Sympathetic and somatic signals diminish and the parasympathetic system takes control, inducing detrusor contraction and relaxation of the bladder neck and the pelvic floor, and most importantly the active relaxation of the striated muscle of the external sphincter. The bladder empties promptly unless there is obstruction to the outflow. Thus it can be seen that although filling and maintenance of continence are unconscious reflex actions, the urge to empty can be controlled to an extent by conscious action through increased contraction of the striated muscled external urethral sphincter.

# 2. IMAGING MODALITIES USED FOR ASSESSMENT OF THE BLADDER

- PLAIN RADIOGRAPH
- INTRAVENOUS UROGRAM
- CYSTOGRAPHY
- ULTRASOUND OF THE BLADDER
- COMPUTED TOMOGRAPHY
- MAGNETIC RESONANCE IMAGING
- LOWER TRACT URODYNAMICS
  Uroflowmetry
  Ultrasound cystodynamogram
  Videourodynamics

## PLAIN ABDOMINAL RADIOGRAPH

Prior to the introduction of ultrasound, the plain abdominal radiograph or the 'KUB (kidney, ureter, bladder)', followed by an intravenous (IVU) or excretory (EU) urogram, was the 'workhorse' imaging modality of the urinary tract. Its use is now increasingly challenged by the explosion in the technical ability of the cross-sectional and computerised modalities, such as ultrasound, computerised tomography (CT) and magnetic resonance imaging (MRI), however, it still retains a role in certain situations. Its particular value is in demonstrating the presence or absence of calcification or calculi related to the urogenital tract (Figure 2.1).

For confident imaging it is important to ensure that the entire tract is imaged adequately, from the upper poles of the kidneys to the bladder base, and further supplementary views may be necessary. Oblique views, views in another phase of respiration or plain tomography can all contribute to improved visualisation of the renal areas and increase diagnostic confidence. However, additional views, e.g. oblique, etc., do not contribute any further to the evaluation of suspected bladder calcification unless they are taken as part of a contrast-enhanced series. On lateral views, the pubic bones lie over the bladder. The bones should be scrutinised for congenital vertebral anomalies, such as widened pubis symphysis seen with bladder exstrophy and destructive bony lesions in adults of an appropriate age group that indicate malignant or infective bony disease, and a neural cause for bladder dysfunction. The bladder outline itself is poorly visualised as there is insufficient fat surrounding the bladder to confer visibility by virtue of a density gradient, unlike the kidneys and their abundant surrounding retroperitoneal fat.

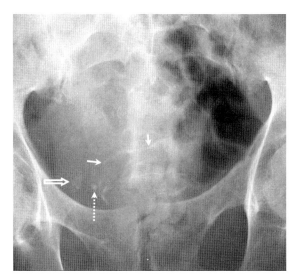

Figure 2.1 A plain radiograph showing layers of calcification within the bladder (short arrows). This proved to be calcified bladder carcinoma. The plain radiograph has the highest sensitivity (after computerized tomography) for identification of calcification within the urinary tract. However, calcification should be differentiated from other causes of pelvic calcification, such as phleboliths (hatched arrow), ovarian or uterine calcification and calcium in arteries or lymph nodes (open arrow)

## INTRAVENOUS UROGRAM

Intravenous, sometimes also called excretory, urography was first introduced into radiological practice in the mid-1900s and the technique has changed very little over the intervening years. Although it is principally a method for imaging the upper tract anatomy, it also gives some indication of bladder anatomy and abnormality. The early images are dedicated to the study of the upper urinary tract, but later views will show gradual opacification of the bladder. Unfortunately, full distension of the bladder takes time and views are not as informative as those obtained by retrograde cystography. Nevertheless, there are many conditions that can potentially be seen on these 'bladder' views but the study suffers from having large 'blind' areas – the anterior and posterior bladder walls are not seen – consequently the false-negative rate is appreciable. Comparative studies in patients presenting with macroscopic haematuria have shown accuracy rates of 26–80% for the diagnosis of bladder cancer (Figure 2.2). The use of the IVU for imaging of the lower urinary tract is now very limited.

## CYSTOGRAPHY

In comparison with the intravenous urogram this equally ancient, contrast-based study still retains a central role in evaluation of the lower urinary tract. Cystography is the fluoroscopic study of the well-distended bladder (Figure 2.3). It is an invasive study that requires instrumentation or catheterisation of the ure-

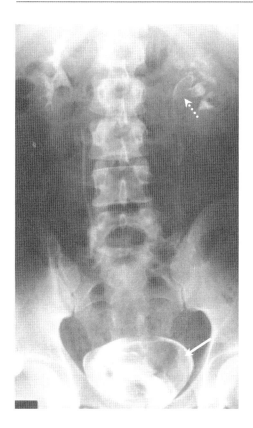

Figure 2.2 An intravenous urogram taken in a patient with haematuria, originating from the left kidney. Clot can be seen in the bladder (arrow) and also in the left ureter and renal pelvis (hatched arrow). Clot in the bladder is typically large and smooth in outline, and usually fills the bladder but the appearances are otherwise non-specific

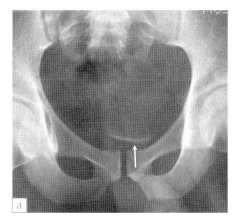

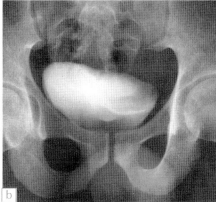

Figure 2.3 A plain radiograph (a) and accompanying cystogram (b) in a patient with thin mural calcification (arrow) due to schistosomiasis

thra or bladder, using an aseptic technique. During this study the bladder can be evaluated for any areas of thickening, e.g. trabeculation, or any structural abnormalities, such as a diverticulum. Intravesical or mural abnormalities are seen as filling defects within the pool of contrast, and stones (or foreign bodies) are recognised by their mobility. Reflux up the ureters, the consequence of either abnormal ureteral insertion, as seen with reflux nephropathy, or the result of widened, incompetent ureteral tunnels, as a consequence of long-standing high-pressure voiding, can be recognised.

The study has similar limitations to the intravenous urogram, i.e. its inability to visualise the whole bladder, particularly the posterior wall. Oblique views are easily carried out with an interactive study such as cystography but views are still limited and this limits its value when compared to the cross-sectional modalities such as ultrasound or CT. Furthermore, there is no information about the surrounding structures, particularly tumours that may have invaded through the wall.

In practice, the two areas where contrast cystography is of continuing clinical value are the exclusion of bladder leak, either postoperative or traumatic (although CT is more accurate in this respect, albeit sometimes difficult to interpret) and the study of ureteral reflux (although this can be studied with alternative, less irradiating modalities such as ultrasound or nuclear medicine). A further advantage is that it can be combined with a micturating study or cystourethrography. This enhances the ability to identify ureteral reflux, because in some cases reflux is only seen during the higher intravesical pressures induced by the voiding reflex, and furthermore evaluation during voiding provides a 'global' view/analysis of the lower urinary tract.

## ULTRASOUND

### Ultrasound of the bladder – technique

A full bladder is essential but the bladder should not be distended to the extent that the patient has pain. Only in a well-distended bladder can true wall abnormalities be recognised, otherwise apparent focal wall masses or diverticula can be simulated by invaginations of the deflated bladder wall. Supine position is adequate but lateral scanning can help to identify mobile stones, etc. A 3.5–5-MHz curved array probe is ideal. A systematic method should be used; first the organ is scanned axially and note made of any asymmetry of the wall. The normal bladder wall is smooth and thin (the normal wall thickness is quoted as 3–5 mm, and measuring < 3 mm when well distended). Next, the organ is scanned in the longitudinal plane. Asymmetry of the bladder wall is again assessed. In the midline, the bladder neck is seen as a short funnel. The lower ureters and the intramural ureteral tunnels should be particularly scrutinised and both axial and transverse views are useful. Again, asymmetry is important and stones lodged in the ureters can be suspected from prominence of the intramural portion of the ureters (Figure 2.4). Transrectal scanning can also be used to visualise the intramural ureter and ureteric orifice (Figure 2.5).

Table 2.1 lists the technical details of ultrasound examination of the bladder.

## Sonographic appearance of the normal bladder

The normal bladder wall is smooth (Figure 2.4) and any focal variation in wall thickness should be scrutinised for mucosa-based masses or diverticula. Occasionally the different layers of the bladder wall can be differentiated but not sufficiently well for accurate analysis (for example for staging of bladder cancer). Well distended, it is ovoid in shape in the longitudinal plane and quadrangular on axial scans. The bladder base is smooth in outline and the intramural ureters are seen as linear corrugations along the base. These corrugations should not be mistaken for a mural mass. In the absence of prostatomegaly the base should not be elevated and the bladder neck should be closed. Urine is fully transonic, but occasionally the more concentrated urine may layer posteriorly or be seen as an echogenic jet as it ejects from the ureter. Differences in specific gravity may account for this visibility of what is, theoretically, transonic urine (as well as the visibility of urine flow across the ureteral orifices on colour Doppler imaging – Figure 2.5).

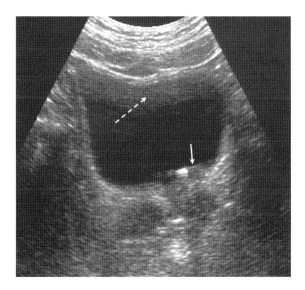

Figure 2.4 An axial ultrasound view showing a calculus lodged in the ureteric orifice. The surrounding tissue thickening is due to inflammatory change (arrow). Repeat scanning in a decubitus position would demonstrate lack of mobility, differentiating a stone in the lower ureter from one lying free within the bladder. Note also the reverberation artefact beneath the anterior bladder wall (hatched arrow), which interferes with analysis of the anterior bladder wall (see text)

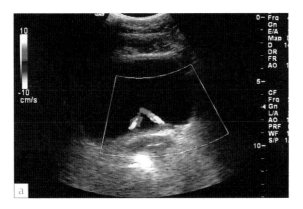

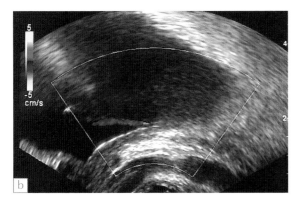

Figure 2.5 (a) An axial ultrasound view of the ureteral orifices and 'ureteric' jets seen with colour Doppler ultrasound. This represents urine flowing into the bladder. Normal frequency is one to three jets per minute, depending on the degree of hydration and diuresis. However, the most important finding is symmetrical flow rather than rate. Absent or slow flow from one side is seen in patients with complete or partial ureteric obstruction. (b) This is a more detailed view of the ureteric orifice and colour Doppler ureteric jet. This image was taken using transrectal ultrasound

The transonic urine makes bladder-wall analysis easy but marked reverberation artefact may be seen and examination of the anterior wall (Figure 2.4), lateral wall and base may be difficult. Suspected lesions of the anterior wall may be better evaluated with a higher frequency probe (7.5–10 MHz) and the base may be better evaluated by transrectal scanning. Harmonic or pulse inversion imaging (broadly speaking both methods remove low-frequency sonic artefact or 'clutter', usually the result of reverberation artefact) helps better to define the wall.

On colour flow imaging the normal bladder wall is avascular but urine may be seen ejecting from the ureteric orifices as 'colour jets' (Figure 2.5). Visualisation of jets is improved by hydration (500 ml of oral fluid intake prior to scanning, though some use intravenous hydration or diuretic agents to expedite urinary flow and bladder filling). Normal jets are well-defined, generally symmetrical cones of colour turbulence, directed anteromedially. Jet frequency is one to three per minute, depending on the state of hydration and level of diuresis, but symmetry is a more useful assessment than jet frequency (Table 2.2).

## Table 2.1 Ultrasound examination of the bladder

**Preparation**
Full bladder – at least 200 ml, and preferably > 400 ml

**Position**
Supine (oblique/decubitus in some)

**Probes**
3.5–5 MHz curved array probe; 7.5–10 MHz may be useful for the anterior wall
(± harmonic/pulse inversion imaging)

**Method**
Scan systematically in both axial and longitudinal planes

**Images**
Axial and longitudinal positions

**Assess**
Bladder wall
- thickness – normally < 3 mm (range 3–5 mm) thick when well distended
- trabeculation
- focal masses – assess location, whether solid/cystic. Does it continue above bladder wall? Does the mass shadow? Is it mobile? (Use decubitus scanning to decide)

Diverticula – location, size of diverticulum/opening, stone/mass inside diverticulum
Bladder base
- ureteric orifices and intramural ureter – calculi, ureterocoele, jets
- bladder neck
- base elevation – prostate enlargement

Scrutinise the blind areas (use harmonic/pulse inversion imaging)
- assess anterior wall using a 5–7.5 MHz probe
- lateral walls – angulate the probe
- bladder base – transrectal probe if suspicion persists

Bladder volume = height x width x depth x 0.52
Urinary flowmetry and post-void residue (if appropriate)

## Table 2.2 Urinary jet analysis using colour Doppler ultrasound

|           | Normal          | Abnormal                                                                                          |
|-----------|-----------------|---------------------------------------------------------------------------------------------------|
| Frequency | 3–5/min         | Absent jets on one side with complete obstruction Reduced jets with partial obstruction            |
| Direction | Antero-medial   | Misdirected with either ectopic ureteral orifice or stone or mass in the transmural portion of the ureter |
| Pattern   | Homogeneous jet | Diffuse or disorganised jet may be seen with high diuresis, or with mass/stone in the transmural ureter |

Note: High diuresis should be ensured by oral or intravenous hydration and examination done with a moderately full bladder

## COMPUTED TOMOGRAPHY

The combination of ultrasound and contrast studies can answer many of the clinical problems originating in the bladder. However, cross-sectional imaging in the form of CT and MRI are vital complementary tools in the investigation of several conditions, and are indispensable for staging cancers. Their particular advantages are in providing detailed demonstration of overall bladder and pelvic anatomy (Figure 2.6). CT, however, has limitations when applied to the urinary tract beyond the bladder. Imaging of the prostate, penis and urethra is better performed by MRI. Nonetheless, recent advances, such as multislice scanning with isotropic, or at least near isotropic, imaging, have further improved the precision of CT.

Isotropic imaging means that the voxel (or block) of imaging is acquired as a perfect cube and is therefore as dimensionally accurate as possible. This means that three-dimensional reconstruction of the contrast-filled bladder is rendered precisely and virtual cystoscopy is possible. These techniques are still being investigated, but CT is being touted as a one-stop imaging of the entire urinary tract to replace ultrasound and conventional contrast studies, possibly even conventional cystoscopy, but this requires further technical developments. Enthusiasm for the new possibilities that these changes have brought to CT scanning must be tempered by the knowledge that there is an increase in radiation burden and the kidneys are subjected to a large, potentially nephrotoxic, contrast load in contrast-enhanced studies, which must not be dismissed lightly.

Table 2.3 lists the technical details of CT of the bladder.

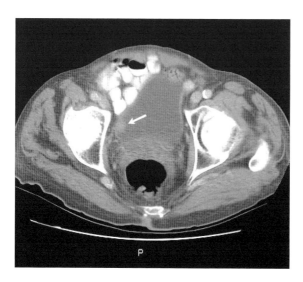

Figure 2.6 An axial computerised tomographic view of the bladder. Computerized tomography (CT) and magnetic resonance imaging (MRI) are best at demonstrating pelvic anatomy and are essential for tumour staging. A mural-based soft tissue mass is seen on the right lateral wall (arrow). This proved to be a stage T2b bladder cancer. Although CT and MRI can demonstrate a mass, biopsy is necessary to confirm its nature

## MAGNETIC RESONANCE IMAGING

MRI of the pelvis provides much better anatomical visualisation than CT because of its inherently superior contrast resolution. In particular, heavy T2-weighted MRI is ideally suited for imaging of the urinary bladder because the organ is fluid filled (Figure 2.7). Relatively longer imaging times have proved problematic in

| Table 2.3   Computed tomography (CT) of the bladder |
| --- |
| **Pre-procedure** |
| Fasting for 4 h |
| Full or moderately full bladder |
| Intravenous access |
| |
| **Procedure** |
| Oral contrast medium for 30–60 min before (with multidetector CT oral water may be adequate) |
| 100 ml of intravenous iodinated contrast medium injected at 3–4 ml/s |
| Acquisition commenced at 60–90 s after start of intravenous injection |
| 5–7 mm slice thickness of the entire abdomen and pelvis (with multidetector CT the images can be reconstructed at 2.5–3 mm slice thickness) |
| Further acquisition can be carried out in 7–10 min to show an opacified bladder but this is seldom necessary with modern scanners |
| |
| **Viewing** |
| The images are viewed as axial studies at soft tissue and bone settings |
| If feasible, reformatted images in the axial and coronal planes are helpful |

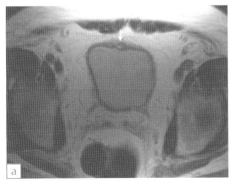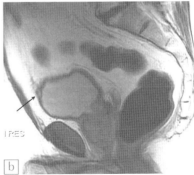

Figure 2.7   Axial (a) and sagittal (b) T2-weighted magnetic resonance imaging (MRI) views of the pelvis and bladder. MRI is particularly good at demonstration of the soft tissues, and on these T2 scans the urine in the bladder has a high signal. The bladder and the surrounding perivesical fat are well visualised. An anterior urachal cyst or remnant is shown (arrow)

MRI but CT is not the only radiological technique to benefit from rapid technological changes. MRI is now faster, with less movement artefact, and therefore has improved image quality and resolution. Gadolinium-enhanced or T2-weighted coronal images can further improve bladder visualisation. The obvious advantages include the lack of both ionising radiation and nephrotoxic contrast media necessary for CT, which is particularly useful in cases of pregnancy and renal failure. The indications for MRI have been slowly increasing over the past decade and it is now used as the standard imaging modality for staging pelvic cancers. Table 2.4 details the technical aspects of MRI of the bladder.

## ASSESSMENT OF LOWER TRACT URODYNAMICS

The imaging modalities explained above are principally anatomical investigations with little useful or direct information about the functional normality or otherwise of the bladder. The bladder is a storage organ, which once full empties down a conduit, much as any inflated structure with an inherent elasticity to its wall and with a single outlet pipe with a regulatory valve would do. Such a structure should obey simple, well-known physical principles, and be analysable according to these principles. Although the concept of the dynamic assessment of bladder filling and emptying has obvious attractions, in practice such tests have their limitations. These arise from the technical difficulties of accurate measurement *in vivo* and the innate complexity of bladder function, which challenges the simple physical concepts outlined above. Finally, there is a considerable overlap between the different

| Table 2.4   Magnetic resonance imaging of the bladder |
|---|
| **Pre-procedure** |
| Full or moderately full bladder |
| Intravenous access not routinely necessary |
| |
| **Procedure** |
| Pelvic images are obtained with a pelvic coil |
| •   T1 axial |
| •   T2 axial |
| •   T2 coronal |
| |
| Other sequences useful |
| •   fat suppression (STIR) images |
| •   post-contrast T1 images |
| •   three-dimensional gradient echo images |
| •   sagittal images |
| |
| This is merely an example of the images and sequences that may be used. The choice depends on the type and speed of the scanner used |

clinical disorders of bladder dysfunction, e.g. storage function can be accompanied by disordered muscular stability, such that it is sometimes impossible to separate the two and identify the dominant or primary cause.

A further, more prosaic, difficulty is the lack of uniformity in the terminology used for the various indices of bladder function. Because of this it has proven difficult to compare published results and studies. Inevitably, many have regarded urodynamics as a difficult, imprecise study with poor reproducibility and of limited clinical value. The work of the International Continence Society has improved this situation considerably and it is hoped that terminological uniformity will help to define properly the clinical place of modern urodynamics. Table 2.5 summarises these various definitions.

## Table 2.5 Terminology of urodynamic measurements

**Pressure**
Intravesical – pressure within bladder
Abdominal – pressure surrounding the bladder
Detrusor – abdominal minus intravesical pressure

**Filling**
Fast fill rate = 100 ml/min
Medium fill rate = 50 ml/min
Slow fill rate = 20 ml/min
Physiological = body weight/4 in ml/min

**Bladder sensation**
First sensation – when first aware of bladder filling
First desire – can void, but can also wait
Strong desire – persistent desire to void, no fear of leak
Increased sensation – early first sensation or first desire

**Detrusor function on filling**
Normal – no substantial change in pressure on filling
Detrusor overactivity – involuntary detrusor contraction, spontaneous or provoked; may be:
• phasic – wave-like, may not lead to leak
• terminal – at full capacity, uncontrollable
• neurogenic detrusor overactivity (previously hyperreflexia)
• idiopathic detrusor overactivity (previously detrusor instability)

**Voiding**
Maximum flow rate – during voiding
Opening detrusor pressure – pressure on commencement of flow
Pressure at maximum flow – lowest pressure at maximal flow rate
Detrusor underactivity – contraction of reduced rate
Acontractile detrusor – no discernable detrusor activity

There are a variety of methods for the assessment of lower tract urodynamics (Table 2.6) and the last three of which are further explained below.

## Simple flowmetry

This is the simplest test of gross bladder function and is a very useful first test in the patient presenting with voiding dysfunction. In many patients with lower urinary tract symptoms, this may be the only test necessary. The test requires a flowmeter, of which the commonest type has a disc that rotates at a constant rate. The urinary stream falling on the disc alters its inertia and the change in force required to sustain a constant rotating speed is computed into the urinary flow rate. Figure 2.8 is the normal flow curve.

Age and sex of the patient will influence flow rates but there are some recognised sources of measurement error. Of these the amount of voided volume is most important, and a volume of $> 150$ ml should be ensured. In practical terms this means that the patient should be asked to void when they feel their 'normal' urge to void. Other sources of error are listed in Figure 2.8. In clinical practice it is often necessary to acquire a number of flow recordings on different days to account for artefacts caused by straining, etc. This helps to develop a reference range unique for a given patient.

## Ultrasound cystodynamogram (USCD)

This test is an extension of flowmetry and further enhances the clinical value of flow rates for everyday clinical management. By combining flowmetry with bladder ultrasound, additional information is obtained about bladder status and the completeness, or otherwise, of bladder emptying. Information about completeness

---

| Table 2.6   Methods for assessment of lower tract urodynamics |
| --- |
| Daily patient-completed volume/urinary frequency charts (3–7 days) |
| •     daytime and night-time urinary frequency |
| •     volume of each void |
| Pad assessment (worn either for 1 h during test conditions or for 24–48 h at home) |
| •     confirms and measures stress incontinence/leakage, during activities such as walking, standing up, walking up stairs, coughing, bending, etc. |
| •     increase in weight of pad $> 1$ g/1 h or $> 8$ g/24 h is considered to confirm leakage |
| Simple flowmetry |
| Ultrasound cystodynamogram (USCD) |
| Urodynamics (simple cystometry/pressure–flow studies or videourodynamics) |

of bladder emptying is important management information in patients with symptoms such as urinary frequency, *pis-en-deux*, frequent cystitis, bladder outflow obstruction, etc. Table 2.7 lists the technical details of this test, with some examples of normal and abnormal findings being shown in Table 2.8.

After scanning the bladder is emptied into a flowmeter, and the following information calculated:

- Voided volume (should be > 150 ml)
- Maximum flow rate (should be > 15 ml/s)
- Average flow rate (should be > 10 ml/s)
- Flow pattern
- Post-void bladder residue (an empty bladder has < 25 ml)

(Note: Voiding parameters are affected by sex, age and the voided volume)

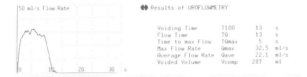

**Artefacts:**

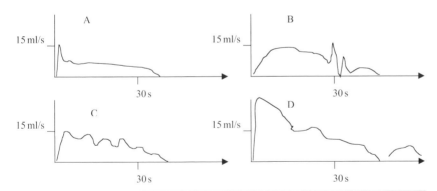

> **Notes:**
> A = Initial artefactual spike due to a jet of urine hitting the spinning disc. True maximal flow rate will be lower than calculated by the flowmeter
> B = Later artefactual spikes due to squeezing of the prepuce resulting in a 'jet' hitting the disc
> C = Wavy profile due to abdominal straining
> D = Prolonged flow inspite of normal flow rates. This is due to an overfull bladder and is often accompanied by further smaller voids

Figure 2.8  A line drawing of a normal flow curve with examples of commonly encountered artefacts. It is important to recognise and correct for these artefacts, particularly after artefactual spikes (A and B above)

| Table 2.7    Ultrasound cystodynamogram |
|---|

Bladder ultrasound for anatomical information
- Good bladder distension is important (> 200 ml at least)
- Bladder wall thickness: the normal wall thickness is quoted as 3–5 mm, and it measures < 3 mm when well distended
- Bladder volume is measured by scanning in two dimensions. The formula used for calculating volume is 0.52 (height x width x depth)
- Prostate volume can also be estimated by scanning in two dimensions at right angles to each other, but it is not accurate
- Distal ureteric anatomy. In the presence of a significant post-micturition residue the upper tracts may decompensate with hydro-ureter and hydronephrosis
- Intravesical abnormality which may contribute to voiding dysfunction (e.g. diverticulum, bladder tumour or calculus)

Functional information
- After scanning, urinary flowmetry is obtained and the post-voided bladder volume is calculated using the same formula (an empty bladder volume is < 25 ml)
- The post-void dimensions of any large diverticulum is also measured

## Urodynamics

The central limitation of simple flowmetry or USCD, is that there are no correlative data about bladder (or accurate detrusor) pressures. Low flow rates may be the result of either outflow obstruction or weakness of the detrusor muscle and USCD may only provide indirect indication of these two entities (e.g. high-pressure voiding will result in bladder-wall thickening if chronic, while the detrusor weakness may be associated with a thin bladder wall). Likewise, in the patient with urinary urgency spasmodic high-pressure detrusor contractions may be the underlying cause. Neither flowmetry nor USCD will identify this condition.

With urodynamics, continuous intravesical pressures and bladder volume are obtained during bladder filling; and on voiding, continuous flow rates are obtained with simultaneous voiding pressures. Such dynamic measurements should provide a more complete assessment of voiding dysfunction, particularly if correlated with symptoms. These are simple cystometry or pressure-flow studies. If these studies are conjoined with intermittent fluoroscopy then the functional abnormality can be further correlated with the lower urinary tract anatomy and structural abnormalities – this is videourodynamics or videocystometrography and is the most complete functional assessment of the lower urinary tract.

It is, however, an invasive test and should be used only in selected cases. Careful methodology is crucial as the test is prone to technical faults. Attention to terminology is also important. The literature is replete with numerous descriptive terms for the various urodynamic abnormalities, a confusing situation that has

**Table 2.8  Patterns seen during ultrasound cystodynamograms of patients with benign prostatic hyperplasia and prostate gland enlargement**

*Normal flow rate – normal ultrasound anatomy – complete emptying*
Seen in men voiding with high bladder pressures against early outflow obstruction as well as unobstructed normal men

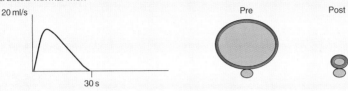

*Low flow rate – thickened bladder wall – elevated bladder base – complete bladder emptying*
Characteristic of bladder outflow obstruction due to benign prostatic hyperplasia. Prostate cancer alone is an uncommon cause of outflow obstruction

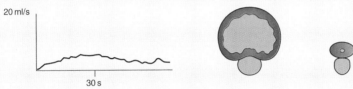

*Low flow rate – thickened bladder wall – elevated bladder base – incomplete bladder emptying*
Suggests severe outflow obstruction with detrusor decompensation resulting in residual urine. Such men complain of *pis-en-deux*, i.e. having to urinate again within a few minutes

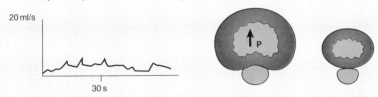

*Low flow rate – normal bladder wall – elevated bladder base – incomplete emptying*
Suggests a failing bladder due to obstruction

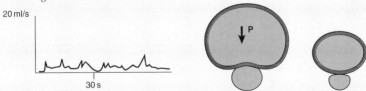

*Low flow rate – thickened bladder wall – large post-void residue and dilated distal ureters*
This is an important combination to recognise, indicating high-pressure chronic retention. This condition can be lethal because of progressive renal failure

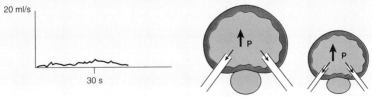

## Table 2.9  Videourodynamics: technique

1. Simple uroflowmetry is obtained before catheterisation, for the free flow rate

2. A 6–8-Fr dual-lumen catheter is introduced under sterile conditions into the bladder – one lumen is for measuring the bladder pressure and the other for filling the bladder

3. A rectal pressure catheter is inserted

4. The bladder is emptied manually and the residual volume is measured

5. The catheters are connected to the urodynamics equipment and carefully flushed

6. The pressure catheters are normalized to atmospheric pressure at the level of the symphysis pubis, whether in the supine or erect position

7. Good subtraction from the pressure catheters is ensured. The patient is asked to cough – with good subtraction the detrusor pressure should show a short biphasic spike. If this is not obtained, the catheters should be re-flushed and possibly may need to be re-sited. Care should be taken over this aspect

8. Filling should be at a 'medium' fill rate of 50 ml/min; unless neuropathic bladder is suspected in which case a slow fill rate of 10–20 ml/min is used. Filling may be carried out in the supine, sitting or erect positions

9. The volumes and detrusor pressures at first sensation, first desire, normal desire and strong desire are recorded. Volume at strong desire is the functional bladder capacity, but filling may be continued beyond this level as the desire to micturate may abate when filling is stopped or the patient is brought to the erect position. Intermittent fluoroscopy can be useful, and note can be made of the bladder outline, ureteric reflux, whether the bladder neck is open or closed and any leakage

10. Any fluctuations of the detrusor line should be recorded, particularly if associated with urgency. This may be the only sign of detrusor hyperreflexia or instability

11. Once filling is stopped, the patient is brought to the erect position and the transducers are adjusted to the level of the symphysis pubis. The detrusor pressure in the standing position is recorded

12. On fluoroscopy the bladder neck is assessed. Normally the bladder neck should be at the level of the symphysis pubis or above. Descent beyond the level of the upper thirds of the symphysis, and beyond, signifies loss of pelvic support and urethral hypermobility ('pelvic floor or bladder neck descent')

13. During fluoroscopy the patient is asked to cough and/or strain and any urinary leakage is noted. The abdominal pressure at leak is assessed (as the 'abdominal leak pressure')

14. The patient is asked to void (a running tap in the background helps). The pressure at the commencement of voiding ('opening' detrusor pressure), pressure at maximal flow rate, maximal and average flow rates and voided volume are recorded

15. Fluoroscopy during voiding is used to record the status and outline of the urethra

Technical notes: Good subtraction should be ensured by regular coughing during the filling phase and prior to voiding. Many women are unable to void standing and prefer the commode. As far as possible, privacy should be ensured. Prophylactic antibiotics can be used. In those with a large post-void residue, manual emptying should be considered at the end to reduce the chances of infection. Vaginal placement is as accurate as rectal catheterisation. In those with absent rectum, the pressure catheter may be placed in the stoma, but subtraction is difficult. Suprapubic bladder catheterisation may be used for bladder filling and pressure measurement.

only served to retard the wider application of this investigation. In this book the recommendations of the International Continence Society are used as far as possible. Table 2.9 lists the technical details of videourodynamics.

## Normal videourodynamics study

In a normal study, there should be a residue of $< 20\,ml$ on initial catheterisation, no substantial detrusor pressure rise on filling to a volume of 400–500 ml and no leakage on provocation. On command, voiding should commence promptly and be completed smoothly and rapidly. On fluoroscopy, the bladder outline should be smooth without ureteric reflux and the urethral profile should be normal. Table 2.10 is a list of all the normal values to be expected during urodynamics, and these are further illustrated in Figure 2.9.

### Table 2.10  Normal urodynamic values and observations

On catheterisation
- no substantial pain
- residue $< 20$–25 ml

On filling
- first sensation at 150 ml
- first desire at $> 350$ ml
- strong desire at $> 450$ ml
- no urgency or leak; bladder neck closed

Detrusor pressure
- $< 15\,cm\ H_2O$ during filling
- no contractions or detrusor pressure waves, on filling or provocation (coughing)
- no substantial rise in erect position

Stress (coughing, Valsalva manoeuvre)
- no leakage
- bladder neck stays above pubis symphysis

Voiding
- detrusor pressure stays 40–60 cmH$_2$O throughout voiding
- maximal flow rate $> 15$ ml/s
- can interrupt flow (the urethra milks back free of contrast)
- empties to completion (post-void $< 25$ ml)

Fluoroscopy
- smooth bladder outline
- no diverticula
- no ureteric reflux
- on voiding, the urethra is smooth and widely open

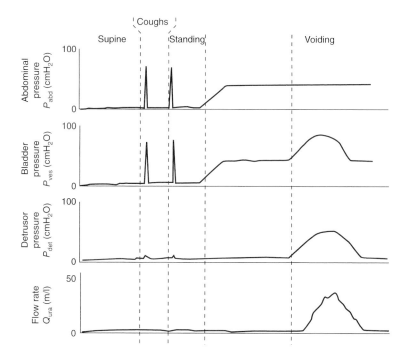

Figure 2.9   An example of a urodynamic curve, showing the voiding phase, with simultaneous measurements of corrected detrusor pressures and the urine flow rate

# 3. Congenital Anomalies of the Bladder

- Absent Bladder or Duplication
- Exstrophy
- Congenital Bladder Diverticulum
- Prune Belly Syndrome
- Urachal Abnormalities

## ABSENT OR CONGENITALLY SMALL BLADDER AND DUPLICATION ANOMALIES

Absent or congenitally small bladder and duplication anomalies are uncommon and are associated with widespread maldevelopment of the lower urinary tract. In absent bladder the urethra is absent and there are usually upper urinary tract anomalies, such as absent ureters and kidneys. Other reported associations include anencephaly and some combinations may be lethal. Equally uncommon is the hypoplastic or congenitally small bladder; this may be a secondary phenomenon as a result of a restricted bony pelvis, or alternatively, there may be further urinary tract anomalies, e.g. upper urinary tract maldevelopment.

Bladder duplication is rare and usually associated with a duplicated urethra as well. However, duplicated urethra as a sole anomaly is more common. Incomplete duplication is rarely seen as a midline septum, which may be transverse or longitudinal.

## EXSTROPHY

The primary fault here is failure of fusion of the anterior abdominal wall below the umbilicus. Males predominate (by 2 : 1) and its incidence is about 3/100 000. The bladder lies outside the body, and in the most severe cases is also open anteriorly. Further anomalies are epispadias, increased risk of adenocarcinoma and, in the female, abnormalities of the labia and clitoris. Surgical correction is necessary.

## CONGENITAL BLADDER DIVERTICULUM

Congenital bladder diverticulum is much less common than acquired bladder diverticulum (see below) with an estimated incidence of 1 : 5000. Congenital diverticula may be a syndromic feature, e.g. part of Ehlers–Danlos, prune belly, Williams or Menkes syndromes. Hutch diverticulum is a particular variety which occurs around the ureteral junction. Morphologically, congenital diverticula are indistinguishable from the acquired variety, both being thin-walled, transitional cell-lined protrusions through the bladder wall (Figure 3.1). Both are also usually clinically silent but they may harbour stones or undergo malignant degeneration (transitional cell carcinoma). Although an increased frequency of carcinoma has been reported in some studies this has not been proven. Urinary stagnation may also occur with a tendency to repeated cystitis. Occasionally diverticula may be large and act as a second reservoir, clinically presenting as a feeling of incomplete bladder emptying or *pis-en-deux*.

The radiological features include abnormality of bladder outline, best detected on cross-sectional imaging, particularly bladder ultrasound (Figure 3.1). In comparison cystography or intravenous urogram may miss a posteriorly placed diverticulum (Figure 3.2). For clinical purposes, once encountered, the imaging priorities are the examination of the internal lining for stones or irregularities. Any abnormalities should be conveyed to the endoscopist so that they are not overlooked on internal inspection, which is particularly likely if the diverticulum has a narrow neck. Second, the dimensions of the diverticulum should be measured pre- and post-micturition. Significant increase in size after micturition may be seen in those with *pis-en-deux*, or repeated cystitis. Such symptoms may be helped by diverticulectomy. Computerised tomography and magnetic resonance imaging can both be used to examine the internal lining; however, they do not provide the

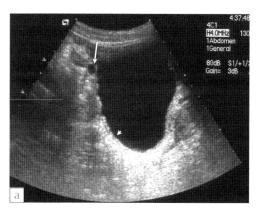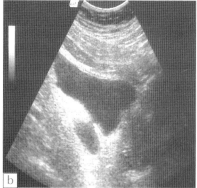

Figure 3.1   (a) A sagittal ultrasound view of the bladder. The long arrow points to a small diverticulum. In this case the diverticulum was acquired, secondary to high-pressure voiding as a result of outflow obstruction, i.e. pulsion diverticulum. The bladder wall is not thickened (< 3 mm) but is slightly irregular. Diverticula should be carefully examined for mural masses or calculi. (b) A larger, posteriorly placed diverticulum. These can act as reservoirs, leading to the clinical complaint of *pis-en-deux*

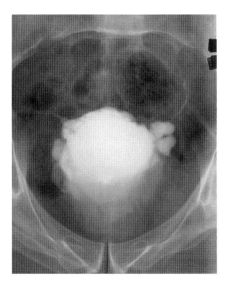

Figure 3.2 A cystogram view demonstrating numerous acquired diverticula and thickened bladder wall in a patient with a neuropathic bladder

ready 'dynamic' information that is available from pre- and post-micturition bladder ultrasound.

## PRUNE BELLY SYNDROME

This is almost solely seen in males at a frequency of about $1:40\,000$. The syndrome comprises deficiency of the abdominal wall, bilateral crypto-orchidism and generalised urinary tract anomalies – dilated kidneys, ureters and bladder with a persistent urachus. Further anomalies may be present, such as imperforate anus and cerebral, lung and cardiac anomalies. The condition is fatal in about 20% of cases. On imaging, the bladder is seen to be large with dilatation of the prostatic urethra; a persistent prostatic utricle may be present.

## URACHAL ABNORMALITIES

The urachus may not involve and a communication may persist between the bladder and the anterior abdominal wall (see Embryology of the bladder, Chapter 1). This is seen in the presence of posterior urethral valves or urethral atresia. In the latter case it is a life-saving opening, providing a bladder outlet; however, this is a rare entity. More common variants are urachal cysts, sinuses or diverticula

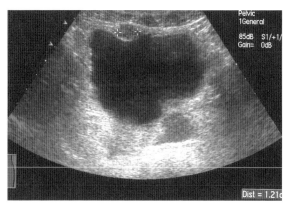

Figure 3.3 An anteriorly placed urachal remnant which (being measured with calipers) is seen to be solid (compare with Figure 2.7). There is an increased risk of adenocarcinoma in urachal remnants and solid remnants such as these should be followed carefully, as cystoscopy may indicate an intact mucosa even in the presence of locally invasive carcinoma

(Figures 2.7 and 3.3). A urachal cyst may remain undetected unless it is palpable or becomes infected. Similarly, a urachal diverticulum may remain asymptomatic as it is seldom large, but it may be noted during ultrasonography. More serious consequences of urachal cysts or diverticula are malignancies. These are much less common than transitional cell carcinoma and are characteristically adenocarcinoma. The diagnosis should be suspected in all anteriorly placed bladder tumours, particularly if there is a prominent extravesical component. Calcification is also proportionately more common with urachal carcinomas than transitional cell carcinomas.

Urachal anomalies are generally noted on cross-sectional imaging as cystic or solid masses located anteriorly within or just outside the bladder wall. The internal content should be carefully studied and any solid component should be examined further by endoscopy or kept under surveillance with repeated imaging. Any enlargement should prompt a biopsy to exclude malignancy.

# 4.   INTRALUMINAL ABNORMALITIES OF THE BLADDER

- STONES
- BLOOD CLOT OR HAEMORRHAGE
- GAS IN THE BLADDER
- FOREIGN BODIES

---

A true intravesical abnormality that is not attached to the bladder wall, is an uncommon finding (apart from bladder calculi) and should be differentiated from a mass or abnormality arising from the bladder wall. This is best confirmed by ensuring that the abnormality is mobile, by asking the patient to move to an alternative position.

## STONES

Bladder calculi may have formed within the bladder or migrated from the kidney. Bladder stones are more common in patients with intravesical foreign bodies (i.e. bladder catheter or ureteric stent), patients with urinary stasis (e.g. those with bladder retention or diverticula) or infection with urea-splitting organisms such as *Proteus* spp. Patients with neurogenic bladders are also at high risk of developing bladder calculi, and the incidence is estimated at between 10 and 15%. Stasis is the dominant predisposing factor, but indwelling catheters, infection and immobilization hypercalciuria also play a role. Most bladder calculi are radio-opaque and are visible on plain radiography, however, faintly opacified stones may be overlooked or mistaken for bowel shadowing. Small stones may be mistaken for phleboliths, particularly if they are within a laterally placed diverticulum or in the ureteric orifice.

On ultrasound, bladder calculi are easily recognised, as long as the bladder is well distended, by their echogenic, shadow-casting appearance (Figures 4.1 and 4.2). Their mobile nature is confirmatory and the 'twinkle' artefact may be seen (these are spurious 'vascular' signals seen immediately behind the stone on colour Doppler ultrasound (Figure 4.2)), which may be related to stone hardness and therefore more common with oxalate stones (Figure 4.3). Occasionally, a stone may be associated with infection or blood clot. A clot would also be mobile, but it lies in the dependent portions and the twinkling artefact is absent. Stones lodged in the ureteric orifice will not be mobile and should not be mistaken for a calcified

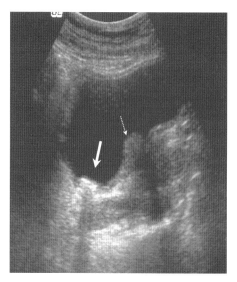

Figure 4.1 A bladder calculus seen on ultrasound (thick arrow), with a posterior acoustic shadow. This is mobile, unlike a calculus in the ureteric orifice (compare with Figure 2.4). Bladder calculi are more common in patients with bladder outflow obstruction, and the hatched arrow points to a degree of prostate hyperplasia in this patient with outflow obstruction

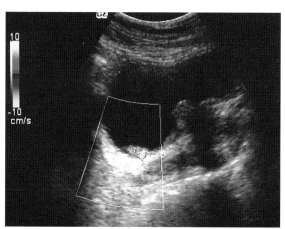

Figure 4.2 This is the same patient as seen in Figure 4.1. Bladder calculi result in spurious 'colour' signals behind the stone, and the use of colour Doppler, as an adjunct to ordinary grey-scale ultrasound, can help to confirm a suspected calculus

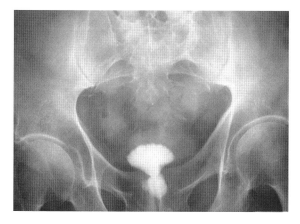

Figure 4.3 A large bladder calculus seen on a plain radiograph. The shape conforms to the shape of the defect left after transurethral resection of the prostate. Commonly, bladder calculi are round or oval, and may be laminated on radiography

tumour. On computerised tomography (CT) calculi are well demonstrated what-ever their composition (except for drug-related calculi such as indinavir stones) (Figure 4.4).

## BLOOD CLOT OR HAEMORRHAGE

There are many causes of haemorrhage into the bladder (Figure 4.2), but the main clinical feature is macroscopic haematuria and only rarely is the haemorrhage suf-ficient to cause acute generalised circulatory compromise. However, acute urinary retention by clot obstruction is sometimes seen. The causes are listed in Table 4.1.

On cystography, a blood clot looks the same as any other cause of an intraves-ical mass (Figure 4.5). On ultrasound, it is usually seen as a variably echogenic mobile layer in the dependent portion of the bladder. A smooth echogenic rim may be seen and layers of hyper- and hypoechogenicity have been described. Occasionally it may be adherent to the wall and indistinguishable from a bladder tumour (Figure 4.6). This can present diagnostic difficulty. In theory, Doppler ultrasound should be able to resolve the issue as haematoma should be avascular but in practice, colour Doppler is not always useful, as signals from true bladder tumours are also often weak. Similar difficulties apply with CT and all cases with a suspected bladder clot should be evaluated cystoscopically, unless there are sound

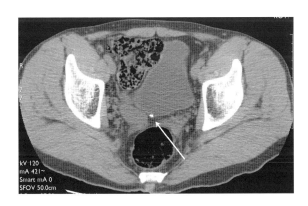

Figure 4.4 Axial computer-ised tomography view showing a bladder calculus lying free within the bladder

| Table 4.1 Causes of bladder haemorrhage | |
| --- | --- |
| Cystitis | Anticoagulation therapy |
| Calculi | Radiation cystitis |
| Tumour | Chemotherapy |

reasons for suspecting an alternative diagnosis, such as chemical cystitis. Even then bladder ultrasound should be repeated after an interval to document clearance of the adherent clot and normalisation of the bladder lumen should be confirmed.

## GAS IN THE BLADDER

Numerically, intravesical gas or air is very common after any lower tract instrumentation or endoscopy. This is of no clinical consequence and does not require any further imaging or treatment. In comparison non-iatrogenic air is rare but

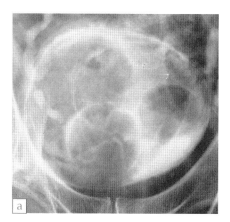
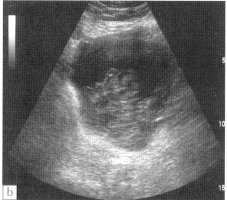

Figure 4.5 Cystographic (a) and ultrasonographic (b) views of a bladder clot, in two separate patients. The appearances are non-specific and bladder tumour cannot be excluded from these views. Cystoscopy or repeat ultrasound is necessary. Colour Doppler ultrasound is not reliable because some tumours are poorly vascularised

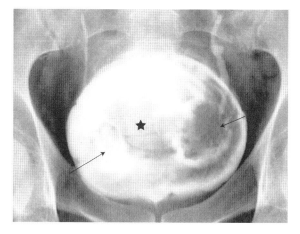

Figure 4.6 Cystographic views as part of an intravenous urogram showing two bladder tumours (arrows). Note that the tumour on the patient's left is irregular in outline and has the typical appearance of a polypoid bladder cancer, whereas the tumour on the patient's right is smooth-walled and not easily distinguishable from the bladder clot (star) caused by the tumours

almost always of clinical importance. The commonest cause in this case is an enterovesical or vesicovaginal fistula, but a rare and clinically important cause is emphysematous cystitis (Table 4.2).

Enterovesical fistula are usually of the colovesical type and the commonest cause is diverticular disease of the sigmoid colon. Other causes are Crohn's disease of the large or small bowel, colonic carcinoma or post-radiation effects. The patient usually presents with pneumaturia and can prove a diagnostic challenge. Intravesical air is usually small in volume and is not generally seen on plain radiography. Ultrasound may identify the air as an anteriorly located, highly reflectile interface. The most sensitive imaging technique for intravesical air is pelvic CT and the presence of air virtually confirms the presence of a fistula in a non-instrumented patient. Visualisation of the fistula itself is a more difficult matter. CT may indirectly demonstrate the fistula if an abnormal bowel loop is seen closely applied to a focally thickened bladder wall. Studies have shown that both barium enema and cystography are poor at demonstrating the fistula. The authors' preference is to perform CT as a first investigation in all patients with pneumaturia. Further investigations are directed by the findings of the CT. In most, the next investigation is a barium enema or colonoscopy to confirm diverticular disease and exclude colonic tumour.

Emphysematous cystitis is associated with both intravesical and intramural air – the air is carbon dioxide produced by bacterial fermentation. This condition denotes severe infection. It is more common with diabetes mellitus, indwelling catheters, or outflow obstruction. *Escherichia coli* is the commonest cause, but fungi (*Candida* spp.) may be the cause in the immunocompromised patient. Plain radiography (Figure 4.7), ultrasound and CT will all show gas in the bladder wall. CT is best at demonstrating the full extent of the local infection and is the preferred investigation for this condition. A laminated, gas-containing intravesical mass is highly suggestive of a fungal ball and infection.

| Table 4.2   Causes of air in the bladder |
| --- |
| Post-instrumentation |
| Penetrating bladder trauma |
| Emphysematous cystitis |
| Vesicovaginal or enterovesical fistula<br>•    diverticular disease<br>•    Crohn's disease<br>•    pelvic tumour (colonic, transitional cell carcinoma, cervical)<br>•    post-radiation |

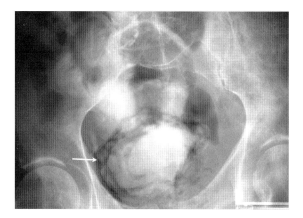

Figure 4.7 A plain radiograph showing emphysematous cystitis. The arrow points to gas within the bladder wall. This condition is the result of infection and is more common in diabetic patients

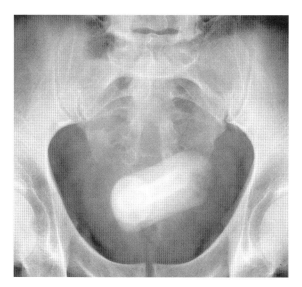

Figure 4.8 A plain radiograph showing a calcified broken urinary catheter fragment. Foreign bodies in the bladder or urethra are prone to calcification

## FOREIGN BODIES

Foreign bodies may be introduced into the bladder deliberately or as an iatrogenic accident. Whatever the origin all are highly prone to calcification and progression to larger and substantial calculi. Of the iatrogenic foreign bodies, broken pieces of bladder catheter or ureteric stents are commonest (Figure 4.8). On imaging they are usually seen as echogenic structures; however, on ultrasound they may be adherent and unexpectedly immobile. Catheter fragments may be missed on CT if they are poorly opaque.

# 5. ABNORMALITIES OF THE BLADDER WALL OR MURAL ABNORMALITIES

- BLADDER WALL THICKENING
- BLADDER WALL CALCIFICATION
- INFECTION (OR CYSTITIS)
  Acute cystitis
  Haemorrhagic cystitis
  Schistosomiasis
  Tuberculosis
  Chronic cystitis
- CYSTITIS CYSTICA OR GLANDULARIS
- MALAKOPLAKIA
- ENDOMETRIOSIS
- RADIATION CYSTITIS
- MISCELLANEOUS
- BLADDER TUMOURS
  Benign
  Malignant

## BLADDER WALL THICKENING

The thickness of the bladder will vary according to its distension. In a normal bladder, the wall decreases in thickness until it is half full (200–250 ml), and then stays more or less constant. Its range is 3–5 mm but with a full bladder it should be smooth and measure < 3 mm. Chronic diffuse thickening of the bladder is usually the result of muscular hypertrophy; a compensatory phenomenon secondary to significant outflow obstruction (e.g. as a result of prostatomegaly or urethral stricture) or occurring with a neurogenic bladder. The thickening may be so extreme as to be visible even with a moderately or poorly filled bladder. Other features associated with a thick-walled, high-pressure bladder are a trabeculated outline (Figure 5.1), pulsion diverticula (Figure 3.2), which are often small and numerous but there may be one or two large out-pouchings, and single or numerous calculi may also be seen. The lower ureters may be seen dilated if there has been decompensation of the upper tracts with transmission of the elevated bladder pressures, resulting in hydronephrosis (see Table 2.7). Correlation with flowmetry and bladder volume is important and this topic is further covered in Chapter 8.

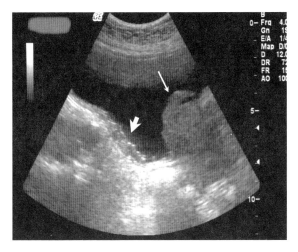

Figure 5.1 A sagittal sonographic view of the bladder demonstrating bladder wall thickening (thick arrow) secondary to outflow obstruction, as a result of prostate enlargement (thin arrow)

| Table 5.1 Causes of bladder wall calcification | |
| --- | --- |
| Tuberculosis | Post-chemotherapy (cyclophosphamide, mitomycin) |
| Schistosomiasis | |
| Transitional cell carcinoma | Amyloidosis |
| Squamous cell carcinoma | Klippel–Trenaunay syndrome |
| Post-radiation therapy | |

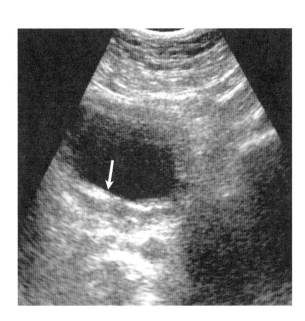

Figure 5.2 An ultrasound view of thin bladder wall calcification in a patient after radiotherapy for bladder cancer (arrow). Thin calcification is easily missed as it may not necessarily cast a shadow (compare with Figure 4.1). Note that the bladder is also circumferentially thickened as a result of radiation cystitis

## BLADDER WALL CALCIFICATION

There are many causes of bladder wall calcification (Table 5.1), but it is an infrequent finding, except in the tropics and in areas where schistosomiasis is endemic.

It is most reliably identified on plain radiography or computerised tomography (CT). It may be easily overlooked on ultrasonography (Figure 5.2) and especially on magnetic resonance imaging (MRI). The calcification may be thin and discrete (and so may be neglected), or plaque-like and in other patients it may be circumferential and outline the whole bladder. Worldwide the commonest cause is schistosomiasis; calcification caused by this disease is usually thin but may also be plaque-like. Tumour is a rare cause of wall calcification, < 1% of all bladder transitional cell carcinomas in contemporary practice (Figures 5.2 and 5.3). Squamous cell carcinoma, which may be associated with schistosomiasis or chronic bladder calculi, may also calcify. There are other causes (Table 5.1), all of which are rarer still and have no particular distinguishing features on imaging, but the calcification of Klippel–Trenaunay syndrome is interesting as it occurs within dilated veins and haemangiomata of the bladder wall.

## INFECTION

### Acute cystitis

Ascending infection from the urethra is the usual cause and common causative organisms are *Escherichia coli*, *Klebsiella* spp., *Proteus mirabilis*, *Streptococus faecalis* and *Enterobacter spp.*; with *Candida* spp. and fungal causes being rare. The condition is more common in women, in whom the shorter urethral length may play a part.

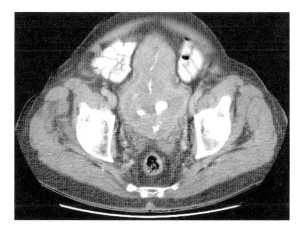

Figure 5.3  An axial computerised tomography view of advanced bladder cancer that is also calcified

Other aetiological factors are diabetes mellitus and indwelling or intermittent self-catherisation, but most commonly they are incomplete bladder emptying and sexual activity. The common presenting features are dysuria, urinary frequency and haematuria, and more severe infections are associated with systemic symptoms and fever.

Acute infective cystitis does not usually cause any ultrasound changes, but severe infections may occasionally result in mural masses (or pseudotumours), and these may be seen on ultrasound (Figure 5.4a). Although their use has not been reported, ultrasound contrast media can be predicted to show enhancement, as also seen on CT (Figure 5.4b) and MRI. Any invasive investigation such as cystourethrography is relatively contraindicated as it is likely to aggravate more severe infection and is unlikely to provide any further information. CT or MRI are also usually normal, but severe infections may be associated with oedema, cobblestone thickening of the bladder wall and marked contrast enhancement (Figure 5.4b).

Severe infection may also result in emphysematous cystitis (usually in diabetics with *E. coli* infections), recognised on ultrasound as a thickened wall with areas of air, which appear as shadow casts but not to the same extent as do calculi. This topic is also covered in Chapters 3 and 4 (Figure 4.7), as it is often associated with intravesical air. It should be noted that sometimes it is difficult to differentiate air within the bladder wall from intravesical air.

In the uncomplicated case with acute cystitis, imaging is directed towards identifying any underlying cause, such as calculi either in the bladder or in the lower ureters (stones lodged in the ureteric orifices can present with identical symptoms of dysuria and urinary frequency), incomplete bladder emptying or diverticula. During and in the immediate aftermath of the infection, the functional

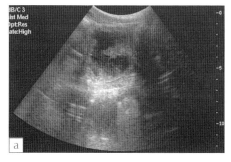 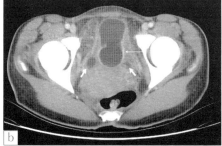

Figure 5.4 Ultrasound (a) and computerised tomography (CT) (b) studies in a patient with severe cystitis. The bladder wall is seen to enhance (thin arrow). Severe bladder wall thickening is seen, and this is causing obstruction of both ureters. The dilated ureters are indicated by thick arrows on the CT scan

bladder capacity may be reduced because of increased bladder sensitivity. This may delay symptomatic recovery but full bladder functional assessment is not warranted unless the symptoms are prolonged and it is suspected that the infection has unmasked an underlying bladder instability. Other causes of continued symptoms in spite of bacterial clearance are associated prostatitis and the 'urethral' syndrome.

## Haemorrhagic cystitis

This may occur after bone marrow transplantation, after cyclophosphamide therapy, or *de novo*. The wall is diffusely thickened and there may be associated intraluminal lobulated masses, but overall there are no distinguishing signs on any of the imaging modalities.

## Schistosomiasis

The parasite *Schistosoma haematobium* infects the urinary tract and is endemic in parts of Africa, the Middle East and Southwest Asia. Entry is through skin punctures and the organism migrates via the vascular system to the muscularis and submucosa of the bladder and the lower ureters, were it deposits its ova. These excite an intense inflammatory reaction with superficial mucosal ulcerations and granulomas, and eventual fibrosis and calcium deposition.

The clinical findings are those of cystitis, but later presentation may show reduced functional bladder capacity. Further complications are calculi and squamous cell carcinoma. Globally, schistosomiasis is the commonest predisposing cause of squamous cell carcinoma of the bladder. Schistosomiasis may be suspected if multiple, or more rarely solitary, focal masses are seen in a patient from regions where the disease is endemic, with evidence of ureteric obstruction or renal dilatation on any of the cross-sectional modalities. The commonest sign is bladder wall thickening, which may be diffuse and rarely the wall may be calcified (Figure 2.3). All these signs improve with chemotherapy, even the calcification, but cystoscopy should be considered to exclude squamous cell carcinoma, as these may also be calcified.

## Tuberculosis

Tuberculosis of the bladder is much less common than that of the upper tracts. Eventually the bladder may be infected and multiple mural nodules may be seen. Chronic tuberculosis of the bladder manifests as a shrunken, small bladder. These appearances are not unique but tuberculosis is more likely if there is also evidence of upper tract abnormality, particularly ureteric and calyceal strictures, although these features may also be seen with schistosomiasis.

## Chronic inflammation or infiltration

There are a number of further causes of chronic cystitis (as well as those discussed individually in this chapter), as listed in Table 5.2. There are no particular or distinguishing diagnostic features to any of these conditions on imaging. They may present with functional bladder abnormalities (Chapter 8), and this particularly applies to interstitial cystitis.

## CYSTITIS CYSTICA AND GLANDULARIS

These conditions are part of the spectrum of urological diseases that includes ureteritis cystica. Pathologically, mucinous metaplasia of the cells of Brunn's nests is seen with cyst formation. The cause is unknown but chronic infection or irritation has been postulated. They are common in women and children with chronic urinary infection, but there is also a poorly substantiated association with pelvic lipomatosis and calculi. The lesions are thought to be benign and, on imaging, multiple small intramural masses are seen that may resemble malignancy (Figure 5.5).

| Table 5.2   Causes of chronic cystitis | |
| --- | --- |
| Tuberculosis | Drug-induced cystitis |
| Schistosomiasis | Chemical cystitis |
| Interstitial cystitis | Eosinophilic cystitis |
| Radiation cystitis | Malakoplakia |

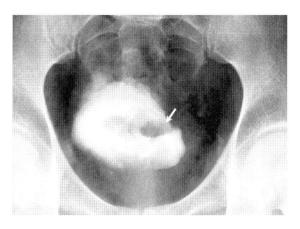

Figure 5.5   A cystogram showing filling defects in the bladder (arrow). On biopsy this proved to be cystitis glandularis

## MALAKOPLAKIA

This represents a chronic inflammatory response, commonly to *E coli* infection. The pathological hallmark is the presence of submucosal granulomas with intracellular inclusion bodies, called Michaelis–Gutmann bodies, within macrophages. It is most common in the bladder and in females of 50–60 years of age. There is no specific treatment. On imaging, mucosal-based masses may be seen as well as general bladder wall thickening, with local perivesical infiltration. The appearance is essentially that of local malignancy but the condition is benign.

## ENDOMETRIOSIS

Endometriosis of the urinary tract is rare but when present most commonly affects the bladder and lower ureter. Patients usually present in their twenties. Pain and lower urinary tract symptoms, including haematuria, may be present, along with a characteristic cyclical history. On endoscopy the mural nodules are typically blue–black but on imaging there are no distinguishing features, although a cyclical change in size may be noted (Figure 5.6).

## RADIATION CYSTITIS

Symptomatic mild radiation cystitis is very common as a temporary phenomenon during and soon after radiotherapy but it seldom presents any imaging findings. Rarely an acute severe cystitis may be induced with diffuse thickening of the wall, with an irregular or fuzzy edge. On CT, increased contrast enhancement may be noted, but this has not been studied with Doppler ultrasound. Delayed radiation cystitis is now very rare because of improved conformal radiotherapy planning but a small-volume, thick-walled bladder may be seen. Radiation cystitis may undergo calcification.

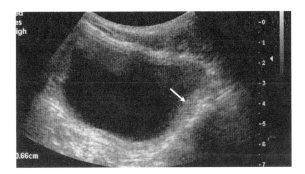

Figure 5.6 Sagittal sonographic view of the bladder in a patient with endometriosis of the bladder. Focal area of bladder wall thickening is seen (arrow)

## MISCELLANEOUS

Other causes of mural abnormalities of the bladder are eosinophilic cystitis (Figure 5.7), drug-induced cystitis and interstitial cystitis. Cyclophosphamide cystitis may be severe and present as a severe haemorrhagic cystitis, and is also a risk factor for development of malignancy (see below). All can present as a thick-walled bladder or a small-volume bladder with chronic disease. Interstitial cystitis is a condition that afflicts women in their fifties and the bladder is usually normal on imaging, apart from a reduced functional bladder capacity.

Further rare abnormalities of the bladder wall are listed in the Table 5.3.

## BLADDER TUMOURS

In practice, transitional cell carcinoma accounts for nearly all bladder tumours encountered in routine clinical practice. On imaging, the majority of bladder

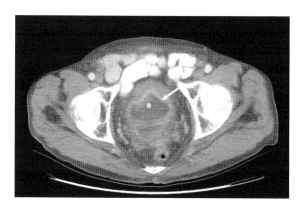

Figure 5.7 A computerised tomography axial view of a thickened, enhancing bladder wall caused by eosinophilic cystitis (on biopsy). The patient has an indwelling urinary catheter

| Table 5.3   Rare abnormalities of the bladder wall |
| --- |
| Metastases of the bladder wall |
| Oedema/inflammation from adjacent structures |
| • diverticular disease |
| • Crohn's disease |
| • appendicitis |
| • pelvic inflammatory disease |
| Mural haematoma |
| Nephrogenic adenoma |

cancers present as focal bladder wall thickening or a mural defect. However, there are other causes of such abnormalities, many of which have been discussed above and are listed in Table 5.4. In practice, it is impossible to distinguish tumour from any of the other causes of focal wall abnormality. Cystoscopic evaluation and biopsy are necessary to confirm the diagnosis.

## Benign tumours

Benign tumours, usually leiomyomas, present as a mass lesion. The mucosa is intact and haematuria is rare. Leiomyoma is more common in women and around the trigone. On imaging it is seen as an intravesical mass lesion and is often pedunculated. Other benign tumours are very rare.

## Malignant tumours

The types of malignant bladder tumours encountered in clinical practice are listed in Table 5.5, of which the commonest are transitional cell carcinoma and squamous cell carcinoma.

### Transitional cell carcinoma

This is the most common malignancy of the urinary tract (around 13 000 new cases per year in the UK) and accounts for over 95% of all bladder cancers in western countries – in regions where schistosomiasis is endemic the percentage of squamous cell cancers is higher. It presents in the 60–70-year age group, with a male

| Table 5.4   Causes of focal bladder wall thickening |
|---|
| Bladder tumour |
| •      benign |
| •      malignant |
| •      metastasis |
| Acute cystitis |
| Cystitis cystica/glandularis |
| Malakoplakia |
| Tuberculosis |
| Schistosomiasis |
| Endometriosis |
| Mural haematoma |
| Nephrogenic adenoma |

| Table 5.5 Malignant tumours of the bladder |
| --- |
| Transitional cell carcinoma |
| Squamous cell carcinoma |
| Mixed transitional and squamous cell carcinoma |
| Adenocarcinoma |
| Leiomyosarcoma |
| Rhabdomyosarcoma |
| Non-Hodgkin's lymphoma |
| Metastasis and local invasion<br>•    lung cancer<br>•    melanoma<br>•    colon cancer<br>•    cervical cancer<br>•    prostate cancer |

to female ratio of 2.5 : 1. Known risk factors are smoking, aniline dye exposure (e.g. textile workers), chronic infection, radiation, cyclophosphamide therapy and phenacetin usage. Over 70% of cases present with macroscopic haematuria, and around the same percentage will have superficial disease.

On imaging they are commonly frond-like projections; others may be plaques or polyps (Figures 2.6, 4.6 and 5.8). Flat tumours are more likely to be overlooked or not identifiable on ultrasound or CT/MRI and unfortunately plaque or flat solid cancers are more likely to be higher grade (grade 3 or poorly differentiated) and invasive than polypoid or papillary tumours, which are more usually grade 1 or well-differentiated tumours. At the other end of the scale (of grade of malignancy or prognosis) superficial bladder cancer may also not be recognised on imaging, as it does not cause any structural abnormality of the bladder wall. Superficial disease can only be diagnosed on biopsy.

The commonest locations are the lateral bladder wall (about 50%) or around the trigone (approximately 20%); but around one-third will have multifocal tumour at presentation and, on biopsy areas that are normal on imaging or cystoscopy may demonstrate foci of carcinoma *in situ* or squamous metaplasia. Carcinoma *in situ* is associated with a higher incidence of recurrent and invasive disease. Rarely, transitional cell carcinoma may calcify (Figures 2.1, 5.3 and 5.9) and dilatation of the distal ureter indicates involvement of the ureteric orifices. On imaging, note should be made of the number of lesions and their location, this information should be conveyed to the endoscopist. Focal masses may be missed if they are inside diverticula (up to 7% have been reported to arise within diverticula, but this figure may be lower in contemporary practice) or in a urachal remnant. Likewise, tumours of the anterior bladder wall or those arising from the base, adjacent to an enlarged prostate gland, may be overlooked. All these areas should be carefully inspected in a patient with macroscopic haematuria to decrease the false-negative rate.

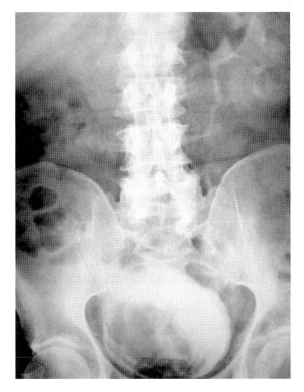

Figure 5.8 An intravenous urogram showing a large filling defect in the bladder, that proved to be carcinoma on biopsy. Note the similarity with benign diseases, in Figure 4.5

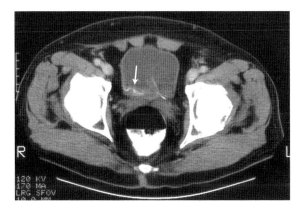

Figure 5.9 Thickened, enhancing bladder wall is seen posteriorly on this computerised tomography view, as a result of bladder carcinoma

The sensitivity of ultrasound for the diagnosis of bladder transitional cell carcinoma is reported as up to 90% and it detects more bladder masses than would an intravenous urogram. However, one study had an 11% false-positive rate (because of bladder wall trabeculation, blood clot or stones – both of the latter should be mobile – or focal cystitis). Small lesions are more difficult to detect and the true-positive rate for tumours < 5 mm in size was only 38%. A more recent study of 1000 patients reported a sensitivity of only 63% and specificity of 99% for all cases of bladder cancer. Consequently, bladder imaging (commonly ultrasound) is not recommended for the exclusion of bladder tumour in patients with macroscopic haematuria, and cystoscopy is necessary in all such cases. Recurrent transitional cell carcinoma is also common, 50–70% of patients with superficial disease will develop recurrence and 10–15% will progress to a higher stage, and surveillance is also better by cystoscopy. However, in those patients for whom endoscopy is not suitable, ultrasound surveillance with urinary cytology has been reported to have a sensitivity of 74% for identifying recurrent disease.

The significant limitation of all the imaging modalities is the inability to identify superficial or early transitional cell carcinoma. It is possible that this will change with improved imaging, of which MRI or ultrasound would be most useful, as high definition CT is likely to be highly radiating.

### Squamous cell carcinoma

This accounts for 3–7% of bladder cancers in western countries. Repeated instrumentation, chronic catheterisation, chronic stone disease (all causes of non-keratinising squamous metaplasia) and schistosomiasis are recognised risk factors. Presentation is usually at a more advanced stage than transitional cell carcinoma.

### Adenocarcinoma

Around 2% of bladder cancers are of adenocarcinoma type. They are almost always seen within urachal remnants or anomalies, however, occasionally, they are

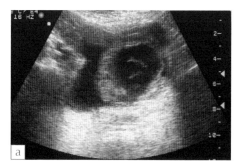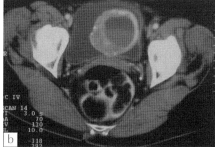

Figure 5.10 Ultrasound (a) and computerised tomography (b) views of an enhancing cystic mass that was a paraganglioma

also found in patients with repaired bladder extrophy or metaplasia of the transitional cell epithelium. Muscle invasion and local invasion are often present at the time of diagnosis, because clinical presentation is often late.

*Miscellaneous bladder cancers*

There are some unusual bladder cancers that are worth mentioning. Rhabdomyosarcoma is the most common bladder cancer in childhood, commoner in boys < 5 years of age. They can be sizeable at presentation and are usually polypoid. Figure 5.10 is an example of a cystic paraganglioma. Presentation was with a typical clinical history of sweating and headaches during voiding.

# 6.   STAGING OF BLADDER CANCER

- TYPES OF BLADDER CANCER
- METHODS OF STAGING
- TNM STAGING CLASSIFICATION
- RADIOLOGICAL STAGING
  Ultrasound
  Computed tomography
  Magnetic resonance imaging

## TYPES OF BLADDER CANCER

Bladder cancer is the most commonly encountered primary tumour of the urinary tract (Table 6.1). The incidence is 6–8% of all male cancers, but is lower in the female at 2–3%; while the male to female ratio is about 2.5 : 1. It is predominantly a cancer of the elderly, with highest incidence in the 60–70-year age group, median age at presentation being about 69 years. The known risk factors were summarised in the preceding chapter (page 44), of which a history of cigarette smoking is the commonest, conferring a two- to six-fold increased risk. Further risk factors were discussed in the preceding chapter, as well as other clinical and diagnostic details of bladder cancer. Of the many cell types that may present, over 90% are transitional cell in origin (Table 6.1), and this chapter deals with the details of staging of bladder cancer.

## METHODS OF STAGING

At the time of presentation one-third of cancers will have multifocal disease and one-third are invasive. Initial imaging may have already diagnosed a bladder mass, however, as imaging is not sufficiently specific, in all cases the diagnosis needs to be confirmed by endoscopy and biopsy. Tissue analysis not only confirms the cell type but also the malignancy is further subgraded into well-differentiated, low-grade tumours (grade 1), moderately differentiated tumours (grade 2) or poorly differentiated, high-grade tumours (grade 3). The higher grades have a much poorer prognosis and greater likelihood of recurrence. The 5-year survival for a patient with a grade 1 tumour is 80–95%, however, this falls to around 60% with a grade 3 cell type. Further information is gained from the depth of invasion shown by the biopsy sample. This allows the disease to be considered in two broad

| Table 6.1 Incidence of the various types of bladder cancers | |
| --- | --- |
| Transitional cell cancers | > 90% |
| Adenocarcinomas | 2% |
| Squamous cell cancers | 3–7%* |
| Mixed cell types (transitional cell/squamous) | 3–6% |
| Leiomyosarcomas | < 1% |
| Rhabdomyosarcomas | < 1% |
| Lymphoma (usually non-Hodgkin's) | < 1% |
| Metastatic | < 1% |
| Direct tumour spread from adjacent structures | < 1% |
| *Higher in areas where schistosomiasis is endemic | |

categories – superficial and invasive. The depth of invasion has a direct bearing on the 5-year survival rate, the rate being > 80% for patients with tumours confined to the mucosa or submucosa, but between 40 and 60%, depending on whether the muscle is breached and the perivesical fat is involved. Depth of invasion also influences the treatment options, in broad terms, patients with the superficial tumour – the tumours confined to the mucosa and the superficial muscle layer – are treated with local resection and maintained on surveillance for recurrent disease, with additional intravesical therapy as necessary. Patients with deeper invasive tumours are treated with the more radical options of bladder resection or radiotherapy. This is an oversimplification of what is, in practice, a complex clinical problem and one that is evolving all the time, however, it serves to make the point that accurate microscopic and macroscopic staging of bladder transitional cell carcinoma is central to the management of this disease. Table 6.2 summarises the staging approach to transitional cell carcinoma.

Not all tumours require staging by imaging. Most tumours at presentation are polypoid and superficial. Usually full resection is performed at the time of the endoscopic excision biopsy to confirm the diagnosis. Such patients do not benefit from staging by imaging at initial presentation. However, on future surveillance their (recurrent) tumour may become more aggressive. It may be of a higher grade, or involve deeper structures or carcinoma *in situ* may have developed. In this case, imaging and staging becomes necessary. Deeper or higher grade tumours at presentation, or those being considered for more aggressive therapy, should all be staged by imaging as bimanual or clinical staging is not sufficiently reliable. For staging, the tumor–node–metastasis (TNM) staging classification is used almost universally.

| Table 6.2 Staging of transitional cell carcinoma | |
| --- | --- |
| **At presentation/diagnosis** | Flat or polypoid |
| | Multiple |
| **Bimanual examination during cystoscopy** | Tumour bulk |
| | Tumour mobility/fixation |
| **Biopsy** | Cell type |
| | Cellular grade |
| | Depth of invasion |
| | Presence of carcinoma *in situ* |
| **Imaging** | Size of tumour (particularly extravesical) |
| | Involvement of perivesical fat |
| | Involvement of perivesical structures |
| | Nodal status |
| | Ureteric involvement |

## TNM STAGING CLASSIFICATION

Jewett–Scott–Marshall tumour staging system has now been superseded by the TNM staging method. This is summarised in Table 6.3 and Figure 6.1.

## RADIOLOGICAL STAGING MODALITIES

Transitional cell carcinoma of the bladder can be staged using ultrasound, computed tomography (CT) or magnetic resonance imaging (MRI) (Figure 6.1). Of the older modalities lymphangiography is no longer used, and of the developing modalities positron emission tomography has not yet been proven to be of great value.

### Ultrasound

Transabdominal ultrasound has poor accuracy in the staging of bladder cancer, particularly in the relatively blind areas of around the trigone. Earlier studies demonstrated an accuracy of only around 55%. Ultrasound is now no longer used routinely; however, there are few modern data available, particularly regarding newer techniques such as harmonic or pulse inversion imaging, or the use of ultra-

| Table 6.3   TNM classification for bladder cancer | |
|---|---|
| Ta | Non-invasive papillary cancer |
| Tis | Carcinoma *in situ* |
| T1 | Tumour invades subepithelial connective tissue |
| T2 | Muscle invasive tumour |
| T2a | Tumour invades superficial muscle |
| T2b | Tumour invades deep muscle |
| T3 | Tumour invades perivesical tissues |
| T3a | Microscopic perivesical invasion |
| T3b | Macroscopic perivesical invasion |
| T4 | Tumour invades surrounding structures |
| T4a | Invasion of prostate/uterus/vagina |
| T4b | Invasion of pelvic side wall/abdominal wall |
| N0 | No nodal metastasis |
| N1 | Single node, < 2 cm (greatest dimension) |
| N2 | Single node 2–5 cm, or multiple nodes all < 2 cm |
| N3 | Node(s) > 5 cm |
| M0 | No distant metastasis |
| M1 | Distant metastasis |

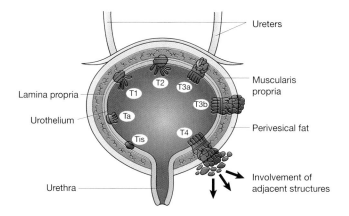

Figure 6.1   Illustration of the local staging of bladder cancer

sound contrast media. These may perform better with regard to bladder wall evaluation but are unlikely to make any impact on the assessment of small nodal status and local or perivesical fat invasion (Figure 6.2). Endoscopic ultrasound is said to be better than transabdominal scanning for the evaluation of muscle invasive disease and an accuracy of 62–92% has been reported; however, this technique has not achieved any level of clinical applicability, being invasive and expensive. At present, ultrasound has no defined role in the staging of bladder cancer.

## Computed tomography and magnetic resonance imaging

These two techniques will be considered together and their advantages and disadvantages will be compared. The technical details of each modality are summarised in Chapter 2. At the moment both techniques are developing rapidly, in particular, much progress is being made in the speed of image acquisition. The advent of multidetector CTs has allowed much faster imaging with marked reduction in the incidence of motion artefact. Multislice technology also introduces the prospect of isotropic imaging, where the unit of information (or voxel) is acquired almost isotropically, i.e. is the same size in all three fixed planes. This allows for much finer re-formatted imaging and coronal and sagittal images may be obtained. Until recently (prior to the year 2000) such orthogonal imaging was only feasible with MRI.

Likewise, MRI has also improved greatly with faster, crisper imaging which should improve further with the arrival of high magnetic strength machines. Thus, the two techniques are joined in a constant battle for supremacy if state-of-the-art machines are compared. It is impossible to be categorical about the clear winner, each technique having areas of better performance, however, MRI has superior resolution of local invasion. Arguably, this contribution to staging is more important than nodal status or distant metastasis. In any case, whichever modality is used it

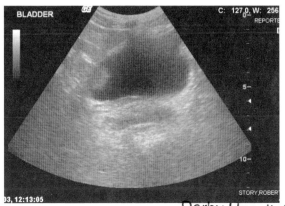

Figure 6.2 An ultrasound image of two bladder cancers seen along the right lateral wall. Ultrasound is of low accuracy for the staging of cancer (see text) as deeper muscular invasion cannot be assessed easily

is important to leave some time after the endoscopic resection and biopsy before imaging, as postinstrumentation artefact is the dominant source of error in the analysis for local invasion. An interval of 4 weeks is suggested, but this figure is based on empirical observation.

The accuracy of CT for overall staging of transitional cell carcinoma of the bladder has been reported as between 40 and 89% compared with 73–96% for MRI. MRI performs particularly well when local staging alone is compared, but the techniques are of similar accuracy with regard to nodal analysis. Both modalities, however, have areas of difficulties. Artefacts as a result of recent biopsy and haemorrhage have already been mentioned. Other problems occur after radiation or surgery when fibrosis or oedema may be confused with recurrent or residual disease. Contrast enhancement with either CT or MRI is of some help in this area.

*Computed tomographic findings*

The primary tumour may be seen as a mass if it has not already been excised (Figure 6.3). In its absence an area of mild bladder wall thickening may be noted, but this may reflect post-biopsy changes. Tumour enhancement may be seen, usually to a greater degree than adjacent normal wall, unless the latter is inflamed (Figure 6.3). Multiformatted images (particularly in the coronal plane) are useful for assessment of the dome of the bladder. In the absence of artefact, wall thickening denotes muscle invasion, but it is impossible to separate T2a from T2b tumours by CT. This is one of the major disadvantages of CT compared with MRI.

The interface of the bladder against the adjacent perivesical fat should be carefully scrutinised. A smooth line of contact in the region of the bladder wall thickening differentiates T3 from T2 cancer. A T3 tumour – perivesical fat invasion – is recognised when an irregular and ill-defined interface is seen (Figures 6.3–6.5). Evaluation may be helped if the tumour enhances with radiographic contrast as this accentuates the interface. An obvious mass in the perivesical fat is a clear indicator of a T3 tumour; and if this mass extends to the pelvic side walls or abdominal wall a T4b tumour is diagnosed. Tumour does not necessarily have to clearly abut the side or abdominal wall – a mass within 3 mm of the side or abdominal wall is classed as T4b by CT criteria (Figure 6.4). Bladder wall retraction is a less specific sign of perivesical disease.

Unlike MRI, invasion of adjacent organs is difficult to identify on CT as there are poor fat lines of separation between the bladder and, for example, the cervix or vagina. Tumour may be closely adjacent to the organ, such that there is no discernable intervening fat line, but without actual invasion. Differential enhancement is sometimes the only clue to separate the tumour from an adjacent organ and should be looked for carefully. Involvement of the urethra is a particular problem with both modalities. The remainder of the study should be analysed for enlarged lymph nodes, and the status of the liver and kidneys. Liver metasta-

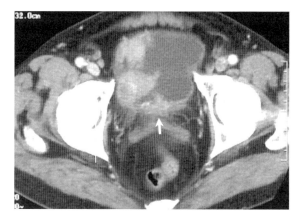

Figure 6.3 An enhanced computerised tomography image of bladder cancer. The perivesical fat plains along the right lateral wall are preserved, although the intravesical volume of tumour is substantial. However, posteriorly (arrow) the fat plains are irregular and this proved to be a stage T3b cancer

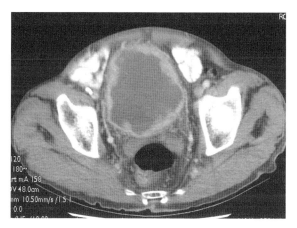

Figure 6.4 This tumour circumferentially involves the bladder wall, and the perivesical fat plains are ill-defined, however, this was a T2b not a T3a tumour. On imaging it is impossible to differentiate a stage 2a from a stage 2b tumour, and differentiation of T2 from T3 can also be difficult. MRI is more accurate than CT for local staging, but comparable for determining nodal status

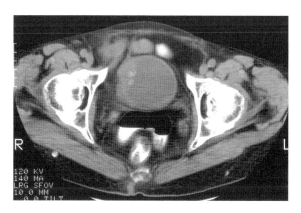

Figure 6.5 A computerised tomographic scan showing a calcified intravesical mass along the right lateral wall. This was a stage T2b tumour

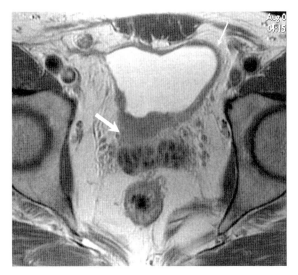

Figure 6.6 A T2-weighted axial magnetic resonance imaging scan of locally invasive bladder cancer (thick arrow). Abnormal tumour reaches up to the seminal vesicles posteriorly and therefore this is a stage T4 tumour. The outer black line is helpful for the recognition of local invasion. If this is intact a T2a tumour is diagnosed. The intact black line is indicated on the left side of the bladder (thin arrow)

sis may be seen, renal metastasis is rare but involvement of the ureteral orifices can result in hydronephrosis and the occasional, synchronous upper tract transitional cell carcinoma may be found.

## Magnetic resonance findings

The clear advantage of MRI over CT is that the density gradient between the bladder wall and the adjacent fat is much greater. This is the case with either T1 or T2 sequences, whereas the inner wall is best appreciated on the T2 studies (Figure 6.6). The individual layers of the bladder wall and muscle are beyond the resolution of current MRI. The primary tumour, if still present, has a signal equal to that of the adjacent soft tissues (such as muscle) on the T1 studies but has a higher signal on the T2 images, although not as high as urine. However, small tumours (< 1 cm) will still be missed. Contrast medium will enhance the tumour and better delineate its margins, although it is not used routinely because of its relatively high cost. Differentiation of T2a (superficial muscle invasion) from T2b (deep muscle invasion) tumours may be possible with MRI, unlike CT. If the outer black line on the T2 images is seen to be intact then it is likely to be a T2a tumour but this sign is not absolutely reliable.

If the tumour has spread beyond the wall it will be recognised on the T1 images as disruption of the line of contact between the wall and the high signal of the perivesical fat. Both the axial and coronal/sagittal views should be searched for this sign. Invasion of the adjacent organs can be appreciated on T2 images. Lymph node metastasis is analysed on T1 studies and involved nodes are either enlarged and/or of the same signal intensity as the primary tumour.

# 7. ABNORMAL BLADDER CONTOUR OR SIZE

- NORMAL BLADDER SHAPE AND SIZE
- SMALL VOLUME BLADDER
- LARGE VOLUME BLADDER
- PEAR-SHAPED BLADDER
  Large psoas muscles
  Ethnicity
  Pelvic masses/haematoma
  Pelvic lipomatosis
- DISPLACED BLADDER
- POSTOPERATIVE BLADDER
  Post TURP
  Post bladder reconstruction

## NORMAL BLADDER SHAPE AND SIZE

The shape of the bladder depends on the size. A well-distended bladder will contain about 400 ml. It is important to measure the volume accurately; either by measurement at the point of maximal bladder discomfort or urgency, or by taking repeated measurements on different days. When < 200 ml in volume the bladder's shape is irregular because of indentations from adjacent bowel loops and pelvic organs. Once full, the shape is approximately rectangular/square in the transverse plane and ovoid or oblong in the longitudinal plane. A variety of shape and size anomalies are possible.

## ABNORMAL SIZE

### Small volume bladder

This refers to a true reduction in the dimensions of the bladder rather than merely a functional reduction in bladder volume (see Chapter 8), and is usually secondary to fibrosis and/or calcification. Table 7.1 lists the many causes of a small or shrunken bladder. However, a small, shrunken bladder will also demonstrate reduced bladder compliance, and therefore reduced functional bladder capacity on urodynamic assessment.

## Large volume bladder

Large bladders with thin walls (< 3 mm) are commonly the result of neuromuscular disease or chronic bladder outflow obstruction. A large bladder with thickened walls that empties poorly is characteristic of high pressure chronic retention and may be associated with upper tract decompensation and hydronephrosis. It is an important condition to recognise as it can rapidly lead to renal failure. A common scenario is that the man with long-standing obstruction and chronic bladder retention is admitted to hospital for an alternative medical condition and is confined, recumbent in bed. As he is no longer in the erect position with the benefit of gravity-assisted renal drainage, the upper tracts become further dilated and renal failure rapidly ensues. On any imaging modality a thin- or thick-walled, large-volume bladder is seen which reaches far above the umbilicus. The causes are listed in Table 7.2.

| Table 7.1   Causes of a small shrunken bladder |
| --- |
| Partial cystectomy |
| Chronic cystitis<br>•    tuberculosis<br>•    schistosomiasis<br>•    post-varicella cystitis |
| Radiation |
| Post-chemotherapy |
| Interstitial cystitis |
| Eosinophilic cystitis |
| Neurogenic bladder |
| Repeated fulguration |

| Table 7.2   Causes of a large bladder volume |
| --- |
| Congenital (thin walled) |
| Prolonged bladder outflow obstruction (thin or thick walled) |
| Neurogenic bladder (usually thick walled) |
| Infrequent voiding |

## ABNORMAL BLADDER SHAPE

Cystography and intravenous urography are the most accurate methods for studying the shape of the bladder, even with their limitations of no visualisation of anterior or posterior anomalies. As these modalities are used less often it may seem that determination of bladder shape is a matter of historical interest, but modern computed tomography (CT) or magnetic resonance imaging (MRI), particularly with coronal reconstructions, can evaluate the shape with enough, and often more, detail. Thus, abnormal bladder shape should be recognised on these modalities, as they can often indicate the cause of the abnormality. However, shape is more difficult to evaluate on ultrasound and anomalies can be overlooked.

### The pear-shaped bladder

This describes a bladder base that is squashed from either side and the shape is of an inverted pear – that is the stalk points inferiorly. It can be a normal variant seen in muscular young man with large ilio-psoas muscles and is more common in Black men. A common pathological cause in contemporary practice is bilateral pelvic side wall haematoma (Figure 7.1) or massive lymphadenopathy. A further cause is pelvic lipomatosis, when excessive extraperitoneal proliferation of fibro-adipose tissue compresses the bladder and pelvic contents. Generally benign, it may be associated with ureteric and bladder outflow obstruction. CT or MRI is diagnostic, but the condition may be suspected on plain radiographs because of an excess of radiolucency around the periphery of the pelvis. A pear-shaped or elongated bladder may also be seen after anterior–posterior resection of rectal cancer. Further causes are listed in Table 7.3.

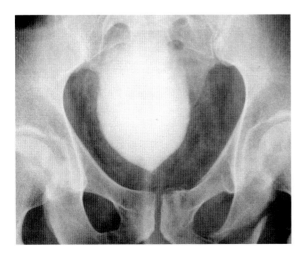

Figure 7.1  A cystogram showing a pear-shaped bladder after major pelvic trauma (there is a fracture of the left pubic ramus). The bladder is being compressed by bilateral pelvic side wall haematoma and subcutaneous emphysema

## Displaced bladder

This is a variation of the pear-shaped bladder. It is a result of a unilateral abnormality in the pelvic cavity that results in lateral, anterior, or inferior displacement of the bladder. There are numerous causes, all rare, but the more frequent are listed in Table 7.4. The main importance of a displaced bladder is that it should be recognised and that, this recognition, should lead to investigation of its cause (Figure 7.2). The mere presence of a displaced bladder is itself clinically inconse-

| Table 7.3   Causes of pear-shaped bladder |
| --- |
| Large psoas muscles |
| Pelvic lymphadenopathy |
| Pelvic lipomatosis |
| Pelvic haematoma |
| Rare causes <br>• retroperitoneal fibrosis <br>• bilateral lymphocoeles <br>• bilateral pelvic abscesses <br>• bilateral urinomas <br>• bilateral iliac artery aneurysms <br>• bilateral renal transplants |

| Table 7.4   Displacement of the bladder |
| --- |
| Lateral displacement <br>• haematoma <br>• lymphadenopathy <br>• iliac artery aneurysm <br>• pelvic masses |
| Anterior displacement <br>• sacral bony tumour <br>• sacral meningocoele <br>• retroperitoneal tumour <br>• colonic tumour |
| Inferior displacement <br>• uterine tumours <br>• uterine fibroids <br>• pelvic floor weakness (or cystocoele/bladder prolapse) |

quential, although it may result in lower urinary tract symptoms as a result of reduced functional bladder capacity.

## POSTOPERATIVE BLADDER APPEARANCES

There are a myriad of bladder operations carried out and thus on imaging many different morphological abnormalities may be seen. Most are functionally and structurally unimportant, but they should be recognised as otherwise they may lead to needless further investigation.

Reimplanted ureters may be seen as focal hyperechoic or fusiform thickening of the intramural tunnel of the ureter or the trigone. Immediately after transurethral resection of the prostate (TURP) an intravesical haematoma is often seen. Later, the TURP defect is seen as a widened bladder neck (Figure 7.3). The shape and size of the TURP defect can be highly variable and have no clear relationship with the clinical outcome and flow rates. Regrowth may obliterate this area (Figure 7.4), but this is not sufficiently reliable to diagnose recurrent outflow obstruction and correlation with flowmetry is necessary (with additional ultrasound cystodynamogram or videourodynamics if necessary), and this also applies to the post-prostatectomy bladder (Figure 7.5). In comparison, bladder neck incision may be barely visible even if there has been good functional outcome.

The augmented bladder may be structurally bizarre, depending on the amount and type of bowel used (Figure 7.6), and peristalsis may be seen. Bladder masses may be simulated by the folds of the bowel mucosa or by mucus strands (Figure 7.6), but there is also an increased incidence of carcinoma after colonic augmenta-

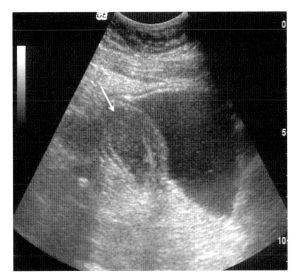

Figure 7.2 An extravesicular mass (an abscess in this case) that is displacing the dome of the bladder (arrow)

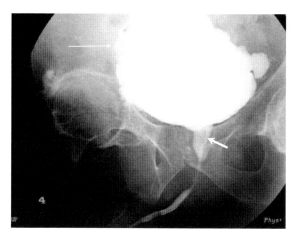

Figure 7.3 A micturating cystogram showing a wide bladder neck after transurethral resection of the prostate gland (TURP defect – arrow). There is also evidence of bladder wall trabeculation (thin arrow) and diverticula

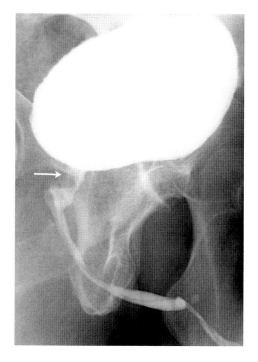

Figure 7.4 A micturating cystogram demonstrating recurrence of outflow obstruction as a result of regrowth of prostatic tissues at the bladder neck (arrow). In practice, flowmetry and an ultrasound cystodynamogram will provide enough information to confirm recurrence of obstruction. A cystogram is purely a 'structural' or anatomical investigation and does not provide the functional information necessary for clinical management

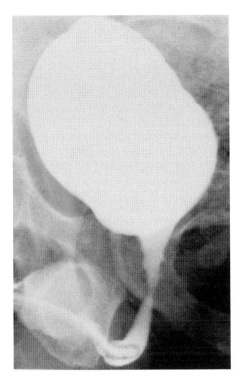

Figure 7.5   A micturating cystogram showing the bladder neck appearance after prostatectomy

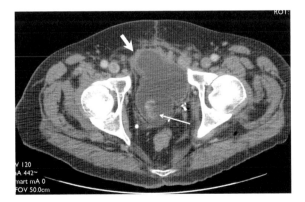

Figure 7.6   An axial computerised tomography scan in a patient with augmented bladder.
Note the apparent thickening of the anterior bladder wall (thick arrow), this is merely a
reflection of the bowel wall used for augmentation. Mucosal folds of 'mucus' may also
result in apparent intraluminal masses (thin arrow). The augmentation was carried out
after cystectomy for the treatment of transitional cell carcinoma of the bladder, this has
now recurred and there is a bony metastasis in the left iliac bone

tion and transitional cell carcinoma may occur in the remnant bladder. Stones are also more common after augmentation and may be seen. Ultrasound cystodynamography is a useful investigation for the augmented bladder, but volume estimation is less accurate, as the reconstructed bladder is of a more complex shape. The upper tracts should also be assessed as the reimplanted ureters, that often accompany bladder reconstruction, may be stenosed or may undergo reflux, resulting in upper tract dilatation or hydronephrosis.

# 8. FUNCTIONAL ABNORMALITIES OF THE BLADDER

- ABNORMAL BLADDER STORAGE
  Reduced functional bladder capacity
  Small volume bladder
  Overactive bladder
- INCONTINENCE
  Stress incontinence
  Urge incontinence
  Mixed incontinence
- ABNORMAL BLADDER EMPTYING
  Bladder outflow obstruction
  Poor sphincter relaxation
  Detrusor weakness
- POST-PROSTATECTOMY DYSFUNCTION
- NEUROPATHIC BLADDER

Simple morphological or anatomical imaging has obvious limitations when applied to the bladder as there is no information about the functional health or otherwise of this structure. In many cases, patients present with functional symptoms, that are the consequence of a structural abnormality, particularly those caused by outflow obstruction or sphincter or pelvic floor weakness. To divorce functional assessment from structural imaging would provide only a limited insight into the well-being of the lower urinary tract. This chapter discusses the various functional perturbations of the bladder and their diagnostic features in functional investigations (flowmetry and urodynamics). First, however, we need to categorise the numerous lower urinary tract symptoms into some broad subgroups to aid diagnostic evaluation.

The patient with abnormal bladder function presents with either a single symptom or a mixture of symptoms, these are commonly grouped together and referred to as lower urinary tract symptoms or LUTS. It is current practice, as recommended by the International Continence Society (ICS – see Bibliography), to consider these LUTS under the broad groupings of storage and voiding symptoms; a further group relates to post-micturition symptoms, but this is not discussed separately here.

Of course, on presentation the patient does not relate that he/she has LUTS, storage symptoms, etc. Rather, they are disturbed by urinary frequency, urgency, etc. The problem for the practitioner is to translate the patients' presenting symptoms into the broad diagnostic subgroups. This will not only allow efficient diagnostic evaluation but is a recognition that the various causes of abnormal bladder function can present with multiple and overlapping symptoms. Table 8.1 lists these various broad subgroupings.

Functional assessment of the bladder still remains problematic. Although videourodynamics remains an apparently soundly based test for a global view of bladder function, in practice this is an area of constant difference of opinion, as indicated in Chapter 2. Of the many criticisms of this test the important ones are that it is subject to many technical errors, not of robust reproducibility, its place is not well defined and, finally, its terminology is constantly being revised. Consequently, it is now used much more selectively. Nevertheless, in such selected cases it is of value in the evaluation of the various abnormalities of bladder function.

Lower urinary tract symptoms may be the result of a number of disease processes. Functional assessment of the bladder when correlated with the symptoms helps to identify the dominant functional abnormality and helps to direct treatment. Table 8.2 expands on the correlation between functional abnormality, symptoms and likely disease process.

These conditions are then further discussed below, accompanied by illustrations of the expected abnormalities on flowmetry and urodynamics. First, a simple update of normal bladder function and continence – the bladder should be able to accommodate a volume of up to 500 ml with comfort and without any abnormal detrusor pressures. At this stage there is an urge to micturate but it is controllable. Any added stress on the external urinary sphincter and the pelvic floor musculature (e.g. by lifting, coughing, etc.) should not result in urinary leakage or incontinence. The bladder may malfunction at any or many of these stages.

| Table 8.1   Lower urinary tract symptoms |
|---|
| Storage symptoms |
| • increased daytime frequency |
| • nocturia |
| • urgency |
| • urinary incontinence |
| • abnormal bladder sensation |
| Voiding symptoms |
| • slow stream |
| • hesitancy |
| • straining |
| Post-micturition symptoms |
| • incomplete emptying |
| • post-micturition dribble |

Table 8.2  Correlation between lower urinary tract syndrome (LUTS), abnormality of bladder function and causes

| Functional abnormality | LUTS | Bladder abnormality | Causes |
|---|---|---|---|
| **Abnormal bladder storage** | | | |
| Reduced functional bladder capacity | frequency, dysuria | decreased bladder compliance increased bladder sensitivity | chronic inflammation, radiation cystitis urinary tract infection, malignancy, inflammation |
| Small volume bladder | frequency | partial cystectomy compression of bladder fibrotic bladder | pelvic haematoma, lymph nodes tuberculosis, schistosomiasis, radiation |
| Bladder overactivity | urgency, frequency | unstable | non-neurological (after bladder outflow obstruction) |
| | | hyperreflexia | neurological |
| Sphincter incompetence and incontinence | leakage, frequency | urethral sphincter or bladder neck weakness loss of bladder neck support | neurologic, trauma, idiopathic age, parturition |
| **Abnormal bladder emptying** | | | |
| Bladder outflow obstruction (BOO) | poor stream, hesitancy (may be associated with frequency – above) | urethral stricture prostate enlargement calculi bladder tumour/mass | |
| Poor sphincter relaxation | poor stream, hesitancy | bladder neck dyssynergia external sphincter dyssynergia | neuropathic bladder, anxiety neuropathic bladder |
| Detrusor weakness | poor stream, hesitancy | underactive detrusor acontractile detrusor | muscular failure after prolonged bladder outflow obstruction e.g. herniated disc |
| Ineffective emptying | frequency, incomplete emptying (*Pis-en-deux*) | bladder diverticulum cystocoele | |

## ABNORMAL BLADDER STORAGE

### Reduced functional bladder capacity

The normal bladder should comfortably hold 400–500 ml. The patient may feel like emptying the bladder but this is controlled. Reduced functional bladder capacity refers to the desire to micturate at a much lower volume. Desire may be so strong as to amount to urinary urgency, and frank leakage may also be a complaint. The commonest cause is the increased bladder sensitivity that occurs during and for some time after bladder infection. Other causes are malignancy, which may be carcinoma *in situ* rather than an obvious bladder cancer. The hallmarks of increased sensitivity are that functional capacity is reduced but there is no abnormality of detrusor pressures (Figure 8.1).

A separate source of reduced functional capacity is decreased bladder compliance (compliance is further discussed under bladder overactivity below). This condition, unlike increased bladder sensitivity, is associated with increased and abnormal detrusor pressures. The pressure is seen to rise $> 15\,cmH_2O$ after only modest bladder filling accompanied by symptoms of desire and urgency. Reduced compliance may be associated with bladder outflow obstruction or a neuropathic bladder (Figure 8.2), or occasionally may be idiopathic.

### Small volume bladder

Unlike reduced functional capacity, this is a true or physical restriction in bladder capacity. The main symptom is urinary frequency. The main causes are previous bladder resection or the presence of a large intravesical mass, or compression by surrounding structures. Further causes are bladder fibrosis – tuberculosis is seen less frequently now but schistosomiasis continues to be encountered. Radiation fibrosis is also less common now with the improvements in delivery of radiation. The functional abnormalities encountered are described in Figure 8.3; note the similarity with reduced bladder compliance.

### Bladder overactivity (the unstable bladder or detrusor overactivity)

A normal bladder would naturally demonstrate normal compliance. It should 'comply' with its role as a storage reservoir easily, i.e. it should be able to store physiological volumes of urine without difficulty. By definition, compliance is the change in detrusor pressure compared to the change in bladder volume. The bladder is of naturally high compliance, i.e. it can accommodate increasing volumes with little change in pressure. The detrusor pressure should remain less than $15\,cmH_2O$ in the erect or supine positions, and should rise in a straight line when filled up to normal bladder volume ($< 500\,ml$). Even when provoked, e.g. by movement or coughing, the pressure should stay steady without any contractions.

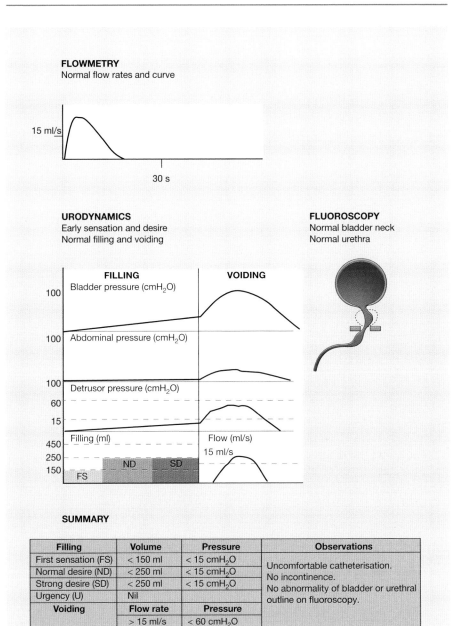

**FLOWMETRY**
Normal flow rates and curve

15 ml/s

30 s

**URODYNAMICS**
Early sensation and desire
Normal filling and voiding

**FLUOROSCOPY**
Normal bladder neck
Normal urethra

**FILLING**      **VOIDING**

Bladder pressure (cmH₂O)
100

Abdominal pressure (cmH₂O)
100

Detrusor pressure (cmH₂O)
100
60
15

Filling (ml)      Flow (ml/s)
450                    15 ml/s
250
150   ND    SD

FS

**SUMMARY**

| Filling | Volume | Pressure | Observations |
|---|---|---|---|
| First sensation (FS) | < 150 ml | < 15 cmH₂O | Uncomfortable catheterisation. No incontinence. No abnormality of bladder or urethral outline on fluoroscopy. |
| Normal desire (ND) | < 250 ml | < 15 cmH₂O | |
| Strong desire (SD) | < 250 ml | < 15 cmH₂O | |
| Urgency (U) | Nil | | |
| **Voiding** | **Flow rate** | **Pressure** | |
| | > 15 ml/s | < 60 cmH₂O | |

Figure 8.1 Functional bladder abnormalities seen with increased bladder sensitivity (which may be secondary to infection, carcinoma-*in-situ* or idiopathic). The striking abnormality is reduced functional capacity (with early sensation and desire) with normal detrusor filling and voiding pressures. Flow rates and fluoroscopic findings are also normal

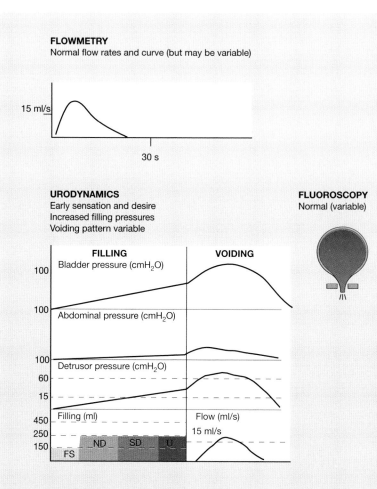

Figure 8.2  Functional bladder abnormalities seen with reduced bladder compliance (e.g. due to bladder outflow obstruction, neuropathy or idiopathic). The dominant abnormality is reduced functional capacity (with early desire) accompanied by a straight rise in detrusor pressure to $> 15 \, cmH_2O$. Voiding (and fluoroscopic appearances) may be normal or abnormal, depending on the associated condition

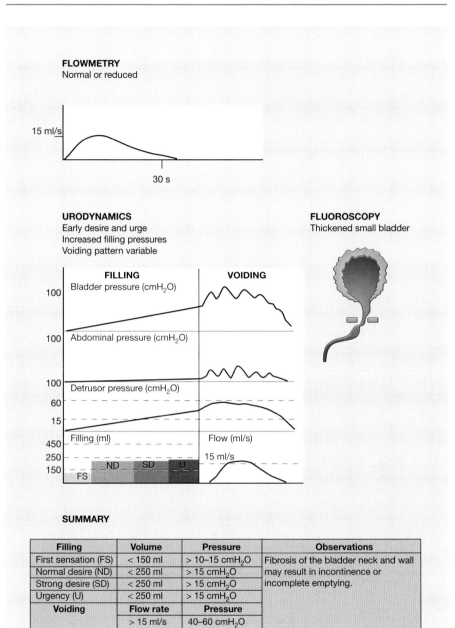

**FLOWMETRY**
Normal or reduced

15 ml/s

30 s

**URODYNAMICS**
Early desire and urge
Increased filling pressures
Voiding pattern variable

**FLUOROSCOPY**
Thickened small bladder

| FILLING | VOIDING |

100 | Bladder pressure (cmH₂O)

100 | Abdominal pressure (cmH₂O)

100 / 60 / 15 | Detrusor pressure (cmH₂O)

450 / 250 / 150 | Filling (ml) | Flow (ml/s)

15 ml/s

ND   SD   U
FS

**SUMMARY**

| Filling | Volume | Pressure | Observations |
|---|---|---|---|
| First sensation (FS) | < 150 ml | > 10–15 cmH₂O | Fibrosis of the bladder neck and wall |
| Normal desire (ND) | < 250 ml | > 15 cmH₂O | may result in incontinence or |
| Strong desire (SD) | < 250 ml | > 15 cmH₂O | incomplete emptying. |
| Urgency (U) | < 250 ml | > 15 cmH₂O | |
| **Voiding** | **Flow rate** | **Pressure** | |
| | > 15 ml/s | 40–60 cmH₂O | |

Figure 8.3  Functional bladder abnormalities seen with a contracted bladder (e.g. post bladder resection, fibrosis or radiation). The appearances are similar to those seen with reduced compliance (Figure 8.2) with reduced functional capacity and a straight rise in detrusor pressure, with an abnormal bladder on fluoroscopy

Patients should feel 'full' but will be able to control their bladder until it is appropriate to void. There is no urgency.

The unstable bladder describes the urodynamic demonstration of involuntary detrusor contractions ($> 15\,cmH_2O$) during bladder filling at a medium or slow (natural) fill rate (50 ml/min and 10–20 ml/min, respectively). The contraction may be sufficient to overwhelm the sphincter tone, leading to leakage or urge incontinence. Most commonly, instability is secondary to bladder outflow obstruction, as a result of prostatic hyperplasia. How bladder outflow obstruction results in instability is still uncertain. Indeed, the basic causes of bladder instability are not yet fully understood, but any cause of bladder obstruction may result in detrusor overactivity.

Idiopathic or primary detrusor instability is demonstrated by involuntary bladder contractions in the absence of bladder outflow obstruction. The cause is not known but contractions may be induced by laughing, etc. Involuntary bladder contractions in the presence of a neurological disease are referred to as hyper-reflexia and are considered a distinct and separate entity. More recently hyper-reflexia has been termed 'neurogenic detrusor overactivity' by the ICS, as opposed to non-neurogenic or idiopathic overactivity. But it remains to be seen whether this syntactical change passes into common usage. Figure 8.4 illustrates the functional abnormalities that may be seen on flowmetry and urodynamics of the overactive bladder, though there is evidence that conventional studies underestimate detrusor overactivity, and conversely it may be present in asymptomatic men and women.

## INCONTINENCE

### Stress and urge incontinence and sphincter incompetence

Incontinence is very common in women and the prevalence has been estimated at 20–50% depending on the method of study and definition. The condition is less common in men (over 85% of patients are women). It is defined as the involuntary leakage of urine, and can be further subdivided into stress urinary incontinence, urge urinary incontinence, or mixed urinary incontinence. Symptomatically, stress urinary incontinence is leakage as a result of any stress on the pelvic floor musculature; examples being physical exertion (accompanied by increased abdominal pressure), exercise, coughing, laughing, etc. Urge urinary incontinence is leakage associated with or preceded by the feeling of urinary urgency in the absence of any recognised stress on the bladder neck or pelvic floor. Some other cases are overflow incontinence or continuous leakage. The causes and the predisposing factors of these various types of incontinence are listed in Table 8.3. Note the overlap with other instances of disturbed bladder function, such as reduced

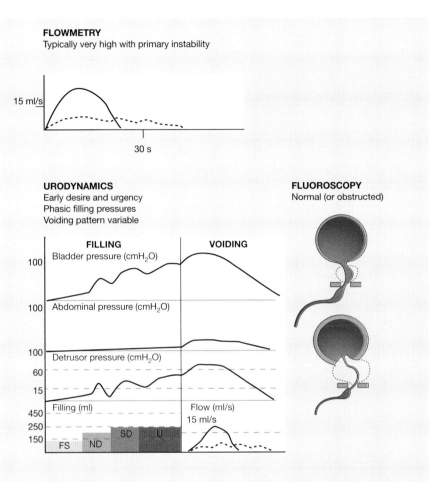

**FLOWMETRY**
Typically very high with primary instability

15 ml/s

30 s

**URODYNAMICS**
Early desire and urgency
Phasic filling pressures
Voiding pattern variable

**FLUOROSCOPY**
Normal (or obstructed)

**FILLING**    **VOIDING**

Bladder pressure (cmH$_2$O)
100

Abdominal pressure (cmH$_2$O)
100

Detrusor pressure (cmH$_2$O)
100
60
15

Filling (ml)    Flow (ml/s)
450    15 ml/s
250
150    SD    U
FS    ND

**SUMMARY**

| Filling | Volume | Pressure | Observations |
|---|---|---|---|
| First sensation (FS) | < 150 ml | > 10–15 cmH$_2$O | These flow rates apply to primary detrusor instability, when they are often high; but detrusor instability associated with bladder outflow obstruction will result in an obstructive voiding pattern (hatched line). Long-standing detrusor instability may result in detrusor weakness (Figure 8.8). Fluoroscopy may show bladder thickness and trabeculation. Strong contractions may overwhelm the detrusor tone and result in urinary leakage. |
| Normal desire (ND) | < 250 ml | > 15 cmH$_2$O |  |
| Strong desire (SD) | < 250 ml | > 15 cmH$_2$O |  |
| Urgency (U) | < 250 ml | > 15 cmH$_2$O |  |
| **Voiding** | **Flow rate** | **Pressure** |  |
|  | > 15 ml/s | 40–60 to 100 cmH$_2$O |  |

Figure 8.4 Functional bladder abnormalities as a result of detrusor overactivity (e.g. primary, neurogenic or secondary to long-standing bladder outflow obstruction). The diagnostic abnormality is reduced functional capacity with phasic detrusor contractions, with marked urgency, during filling. Voiding (and fluoroscopic appearances) will be normal with primary overactivity, but not necessarily with neurogenic or secondary instability

compliance. This further emphasises the often overlapping nature of the several causes of abnormal bladder function; the investigator must isolate the dominant abnormality before a sound plan for clinical management can be made.

Some of the other causes of incontinence are dealt with elsewhere in this chapter, and this section will concentrate on genuine stress incontinence, which is defined as incontinence induced by any activity that raises the intra-abdominal pressure, such as coughing, laughing, walking, etc. A recent document from the ICS has suggested that the term genuine stress incontinence should be discarded and replaced with urodynamic stress incontinence, but there is not full agreement that full urodynamic assessment is necessary for the clinical management of stress incontinence. It is most common in multiparous women and increases with age, particularly around the menopause. The cause is failure of bladder neck and external sphincter competence, when the abdominal (or detrusor pressure) is raised.

Abdominal leak-point pressure is the pressure at which leakage occurs, and indicates how well the continence mechanisms (the bladder neck and external sphincter) are able to resist rises in intra-abdominal pressure. It is believed that those with a strong sphincter but weakened pelvic floor musculature (sometimes also called urethral hypermobility, but this term is less often used now as it is difficult to define) are able to resist changes up to $100 \, cmH_2O$, whilst women with intrinsic sphincter deficiency will leak at pressures $< 60 \, cmH_2O$. Such a clear distinction between the two subgroups (i.e. pelvic floor weakness versus intrinsic sphincter deficiency) has obvious clinical attractions. However, this measurement

| Table 8.3   Incontinence – causes and predisposing factors | |
| --- | --- |
| Loss of pelvic floor support | SUI |
| Urethral hypermobility (associated with poor pelvic support) | SUI |
| Intrinsic sphincter deficiency | SUI |
| Postoperative sphincter damage | SUI |
| Detrusor instability | UI |
| Poor compliance | UI |
| Small bladder volume | UI |
| Fistula | continuous leakage |
| Ectopic ureter | continuous leakage |
| Overflow incontinence | continuous and SUI |

Note that there is an overlap in symptomatology; and many women with stress urinary incontinence (SUI) will also complain of 'urge' because of the fear of leakage during activity with a full bladder. UI, urge urinary incontinence.

is not universally accepted or used, and is a perennial area of dispute and re-definition (see Table 8.4).

Even discounting the many areas of dispute regarding definition and methods for the urodynamic investigation of incontinence, not all women with this condition require full urodynamic investigation. Most can be managed on the basis of history and simple investigations. In those forwarded for formal urodynamics, the practitioner should understand the test limitations and have a clear idea of the specific questions that require answering. Table 8.5 lists, in the authors' views, the

---

**Table 8.4  Urodynamics for assessment of incontinence – difficult areas**

Pelvic floor weakness or urethral hypermobility
- The method recommended by the International Continence Society is impractical for everyday clinical practice
- A more subjective method assesses the relation between the base of the bladder and a line drawn through the inferior border of the pubis symphysis in a lateral or well-oblique view, during voiding
    - the well-supported bladder neck is above this line
    - the unsupported base (pelvic floor weakness or urethral hypermobility) is substantially below this line, i.e. genuine stress incontinence

Leak-point pressure
- Either abdominal (ALPP) or detrusor leak-point pressure
- Measurement not standardized
    - during graded valsalva manoeuver
    - during coughing
- Threshold values not defined
    - ALLP $< 60\,\mathrm{cmH_2O}$ = genuine stress incontinence
    - ALLP $> 100\,\mathrm{cmH_2O}$ = anatomic stress incontinence

---

**Table 8.5  Videourodynamic study in incontinence – main assessments**

Increased bladder sensation
- catheterisation is painful
- desire to void at a modest volume ($< 150\,\mathrm{ml}$) with normal detrusor pressure and no contractions

Bladder overactivity (or detrusor instability) during filling, after filling or on coughing; in both supine and standing position

Pelvic floor descent (on fluoroscopy)

Incontinence on coughing, etc. (abdominal leak point pressure measured)

Any flow/pressure evidence of obstruction

Post-void residue

minimal information that should be extracted from a videourodynamic study in the incontinent patient.

The various functional abnormalities that may be encountered are summarised in the Figure 8.5.

## ABNORMAL BLADDER EMPTYING

### Bladder outflow obstruction

The various causes of obstruction of urinary outflow are listed in Table 8.6. Poor sphincter relaxation is dealt with separately below as it has a distinct pathophysiology. By far the commonest cause of outflow obstruction is benign prostatic hyperplasia or hypertrophy (BPH). Beyond the age of 40 years the prostate hypertrophies and above the age of 50 years, over 50% of men will have some degree of BPH. Both the glandular and stromal elements enlarge, particularly in the transition zone and the periurethral glands, but it can also affect the peripheral zone. The exact cause is not known but hormones play a part. Hypertrophy may be diffuse or as distinct adenomas, and there is also hypertrophy of the periurethral muscle spiral. There is, however, no clear relation between the degree of hypertrophy and outflow obstruction – some men may present with LUTS (frequency, nocturia) rather than significantly reduced flow rates. Others may present with urgency and stress incontinence as a result of secondary detrusor instability (or overactive bladder – see above). Thus, the entire symptom complex secondary to prostate gland enlargement is now referred to as simply lower urinary tract symptoms (or LUTS). As explained above it is most useful to consider bladder dysfunction in terms of the dominant abnormality, i.e. either abnormal bladder storage or abnormal bladder emptying; or alternatively as the dominant symptom or symptoms. Such a functional classification results in a more clinically meaningful approach.

| Table 8.6   Causes of bladder outflow obstruction |
| --- |

Anatomical obstruction
- prostatic hypertrophy
- prostatic cysts
- urethral stricture
- bladder or urethral calculi
- bladder, prostate, or urethral tumour
- bladder or urethral compression by pelvic mass
- post prostate/bladder surgery

Sphincter overactivity
- detrusor–sphincter dyssynergia
- bladder neck dyssynergia

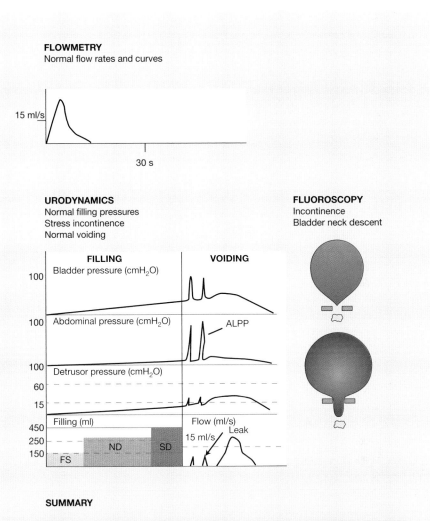

**FLOWMETRY**
Normal flow rates and curves

15 ml/s

30 s

**URODYNAMICS**
Normal filling pressures
Stress incontinence
Normal voiding

**FLUOROSCOPY**
Incontinence
Bladder neck descent

**FILLING**          **VOIDING**

Bladder pressure (cmH₂O)   100

Abdominal pressure (cmH₂O)   100   ALPP

Detrusor pressure (cmH₂O)   100   60   15

Filling (ml)   450   250   150   ND   SD   FS

Flow (ml/s)   15 ml/s   Leak

**SUMMARY**

| Filling | Volume | Pressure | Observations |
|---|---|---|---|
| First sensation (FS) | > 150 ml | < 15 cmH₂O | Volumes (and functional bladder capacity) are reduced because of the fear of leakage. |
| Normal desire (ND) | > 250 ml | < 15 cmH₂O | Similarly 'urgency' may be a result of fear of leakage. |
| Strong desire (SD) | > 350 ml | < 15 cmH₂O | Abdominal leak pressure < 60 cmH₂O seen with |
| Urgency (U) | Nil | | intrinsic sphincter deficiency (but this is an area of dispute). |
| **Voiding** | **Flow rate** | **Pressure** | Pelvic floor weakness may be seen on |
| | > 15 ml/s | < 40 cmH₂O | fluoroscopy. |

Figure 8.5 Functional bladder abnormalities seen with genuine stress incontinence. Filling and voiding pressures are normal, but functional capacity may be apparently reduced because of fear of leakage. Fluoroscopy may show pelvic floor descent. ALPP, abdominal leak-point pressure

For the evaluation of the patient with BPH, the simplest investigation is uroflowmetry or the ultrasound cystodynamogram. The addition of bladder ultrasound can detect diverticula, any obstructing intravesical mass (e.g. tumour or calculus), bladder wall thickness may be measured and other signs of high-pressure voiding, e.g. wall trabeculation, diverticula, dilated lower ureters, can be identified. Transrectal ultrasound of the prostate has not been proven to add any extra information in the evaluation of the patient presenting with reduced flow rates or LUTS. Rarely, an obstructing cyst may be seen near the bladder neck on transrectal ultrasound, acting as a 'ball-valve'. The value of transrectal ultrasound for evaluation of recurrent outflow obstruction after transurethral resection of the prostate has also not been proven. On scanning regrowth (Figure 7.3) and restriction of the bladder neck may be seen, but these do not directly influence management as much as urinary flowmetry and post-void residues. Equally, transrectal ultrasound is not of proven value in the follow-up of the patient on conservative or pharmacological management for known BPH and LUTS. 5α-reductase agents, such as finasteride, can decrease the gland size by about 25%, but this information (i.e. the amount of reduction in the volume of the gland) does not directly influence management.

Thus, in most cases presenting with LUTS as a result of suspected BPH, simple flowmetry with ultrasound cystodynamogram (as shown in Table 2.7) is all that is necessary. However, in patients with indeterminate results, or in those thought to have secondary poor or overactive detrusor function, formal urodynamics are of value. Figure 8.6 summarises the findings seen on flowmetry and urodynamics in the patient with uncomplicated bladder outflow obstruction.

## Poor sphincter relaxation (or dyssynergia)

A normally functioning micturition arc should ensure relaxation of both the bladder neck and external urethral sphincter on voluntary initiation of micturition. Relaxation, however, may fail at either of these two levels, resulting in symptoms of outflow obstruction. Detrusor–bladder neck dyssynergia may be the result of a spinal cord lesion above T5, while detrusor–sphincter dyssynergia may be associated with neurological disorders such as Parkinson's disease and multiple sclerosis. A separate group is men in their twenties to forties who present with a long history of poor stream and on investigation are found to have features identical with detrusor–bladder neck dyssynergia. A congenital abnormality is felt to be the fault.

Similar clinical and urodynamic features may be seen in overanxious men or women with anxiety-related failure to completely relax their sphincters. Undoubtedly, the embarrassment of voiding in public during the urodynamics test will contribute, but characteristically such patients will relate that their symptoms are episodic and much better when they are removed from their particular anxiety-

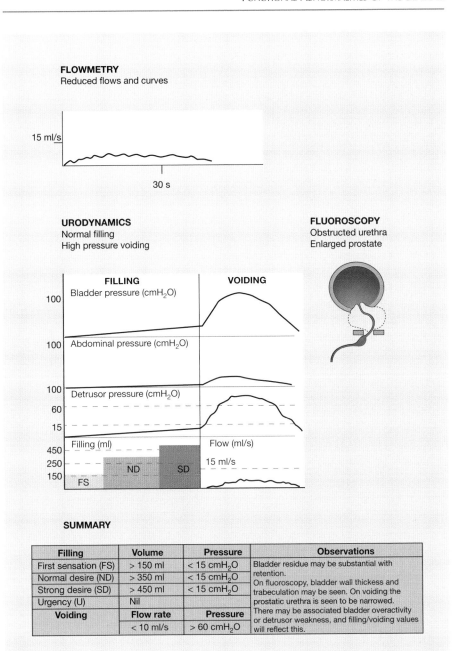

**FLOWMETRY**
Reduced flows and curves

15 ml/s

30 s

**URODYNAMICS**
Normal filling
High pressure voiding

**FLUOROSCOPY**
Obstructed urethra
Enlarged prostate

FILLING     VOIDING

100 | Bladder pressure (cmH₂O)

100 | Abdominal pressure (cmH₂O)

100
60
15 | Detrusor pressure (cmH₂O)

450
250
150 | Filling (ml)    ND   SD    Flow (ml/s) 15 ml/s
FS

**SUMMARY**

| Filling | Volume | Pressure | Observations |
|---|---|---|---|
| First sensation (FS) | > 150 ml | < 15 cmH₂O | Bladder residue may be substantial with retention. |
| Normal desire (ND) | > 350 ml | < 15 cmH₂O | On fluoroscopy, bladder wall thickness and |
| Strong desire (SD) | > 450 ml | < 15 cmH₂O | trabeculation may be seen. On voiding the prostatic urethra is seen to be narrowed. |
| Urgency (U) | Nil | | There may be associated bladder overactivity or detrusor weakness, and filling/voiding values |
| **Voiding** | **Flow rate** | **Pressure** | |
| | < 10 ml/s | > 60 cmH₂O | will reflect this. |

Figure 8.6 Functional abnormalities seen with uncomplicated bladder outflow obstruction (e.g. due to prostate enlargement, dyssynergia or urethral stricture; this is an example of prostate enlargement; dyssynergia is shown in Figure 8.7). The diagnostic abnormality is high voiding pressures, reduced flow rates and abnormal fluoroscopy

generating scenario, e.g. symptoms clear whilst on holiday and away from their job or normal, stressful lifestyle.

The functional abnormalities encountered are illustrated in Figure 8.7.

## Detrusor weakness

This occurs usually after prolonged high detrusor pressures, e.g. untreated bladder outflow obstruction or bladder overactivity, or with a neuropathic bladder. The common symptoms are a long history of poor stream with recent deterioration and incomplete emptying. After a long period when the bladder was able to empty completely, albeit slowly, by generation of high voiding pressures, the detrusor muscle begins to fail. The patient is left with a large, thin-walled bladder. This is the proposed theory to explain the development of detrusor weakness but is not proven. Others believe that these patients are a subgroup with life-long voiding dysfunction, over and above their more recent bladder outflow obstruction. Perhaps a result of developmental abnormality of the detrusor muscle or its nerve supply in earlier life. Distinctive functional features are seen and are shown in Figure 8.8.

## POST-PROSTATE SURGERY DYSFUNCTION

This is considered separately as there may be a combination of abnormalities. After transurethral resection of the prostate (or any other form of procedure to relieve outflow obstruction) the man may re-present complaining of no improvement, recurrence of symptoms, or urinary leakage (Table 8.7). Simple flowmetry and ultrasound cystodynamogram may help to resolve the problem, and will demonstrate if the fault is continuing obstruction (because of inadequate resection or regrowth of the prostate), or if there is unsuspected detrusor overactivity or weakness. Unfortunately, transrectal ultrasound measurement of the cavity left by transurethral resection of the prostate has not been sufficiently well studied to assess the value of this investigation. Available studies do not suggest that is of any value.

After prostatectomy (total prostatectomy) symptoms can be either leakage or poor stream. Most patients have a degree of leakage immediately after prostatectomy that improves over the subsequent months. The definition of continence used in various studies naturally has a bearing on the reported post-prostatectomy incidence of incontinence. If the definition is no protection necessary, i.e. completely dry as is commonly understood, then around 80% are dry. If the slightly looser definition of one protection or pad is used then this improves to around 90%. The main defect is incompetence of the external sphincter, and this is influenced by the quality of apical dissection carried out, whether the neurovascular

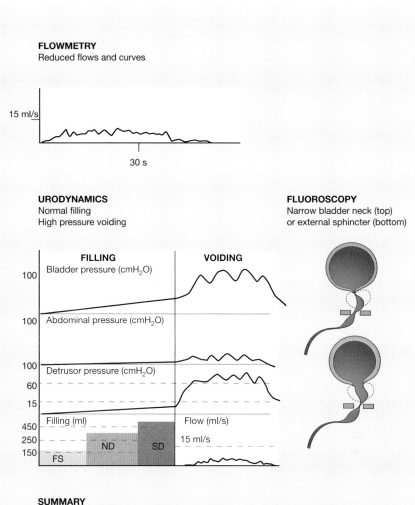

**FLOWMETRY**
Reduced flows and curves

15 ml/s

30 s

**URODYNAMICS**
Normal filling
High pressure voiding

**FLUOROSCOPY**
Narrow bladder neck (top)
or external sphincter (bottom)

**FILLING**
Bladder pressure (cmH$_2$O)
100

Abdominal pressure (cmH$_2$O)
100

Detrusor pressure (cmH$_2$O)
100
60
15

Filling (ml)
450
250
150
FS    ND    SD

**VOIDING**

Flow (ml/s)
15 ml/s

**SUMMARY**

| Filling | Volume | Pressure | Observations |
|---------|--------|----------|--------------|
| First sensation (FS) | > 150 ml | < 15 cmH$_2$O | Appearances are similar to those seen with bladder outflow obstruction caused by prostate enlargement. |
| Normal desire (ND) | > 350 ml | < 15 cmH$_2$O | |
| Strong desire (SD) | > 450 ml | < 15 cmH$_2$O | Fluoroscopy demonstrates obstruction at the level of the bladder neck or the external sphincter. |
| Urgency (U) | Nil | | |
| **Voiding** | **Flow rate** | **Pressure** | Instability, detrusor weakness or bladder retention may be associated. |
| | < 10 ml/s | > 60 cmH$_2$O | |

Figure 8.7 Functional bladder abnormalities seen with bladder neck or detrusor dyssynergia. On fluoroscopy either the bladder neck or external sphincter is seen to be contracted during voiding, which is at high pressures and low flows

**Table 8.7** Evaluation of lower urinary tract symptoms after transurethral resection of the prostate

Poor stream
- continued outflow obstruction
    - inadequate resection
    - re-growth of prostate
    - unsuspected urethral stricture
- detrusor weakness

Urinary frequency
- bladder sensitivity
- bladder calculus
- urinary infection

Urinary urgency
- unsuspected bladder overactivity

Leakage
- unsuspected bladder overactivity
- damage to urinary sphincter

bundles are spared or not and whether the pubo-prostatic ligaments are preserved. Others may complain of restriction of flow rates some months after surgery, and that usually indicates an anastomotic stricture.

Restricted flow rates will be confirmed by simple flowmetry or by ultrasound cystodynamogram, but this will not identify unsuspected detrusor weakness. Further investigation is not always necessary but videourodynamics or micturating cystography will demonstrate the anastomotic stricture. Videourodynamics may be used to study leakage further; stress leakage with an abdominal leak pressure $< 60 \, cmH_2O$ is compatible with sphincter weakness; and the test will also serve to exclude an associated overactive bladder, that was not suspected prior to the prostatectomy (Figure 8.9).

## THE NEUROPATHIC BLADDER

The neuropathic bladder is a generic term describing voiding dysfunction in the presence of a neurological disorder. The condition is best investigated with full videourodynamics as multiple functional abnormalities are often present, some of which may be entirely unexpected. Full investigation is further necessary because bladder function, or its associated complications (Table 8.8) may deteriorate silently (because of absent sensation) and threaten life. Careful lifelong surveillance is obligatory for this group of patients. On urodynamics, a number of abnormalities are seen and these are illustrated in Figure 8.10.

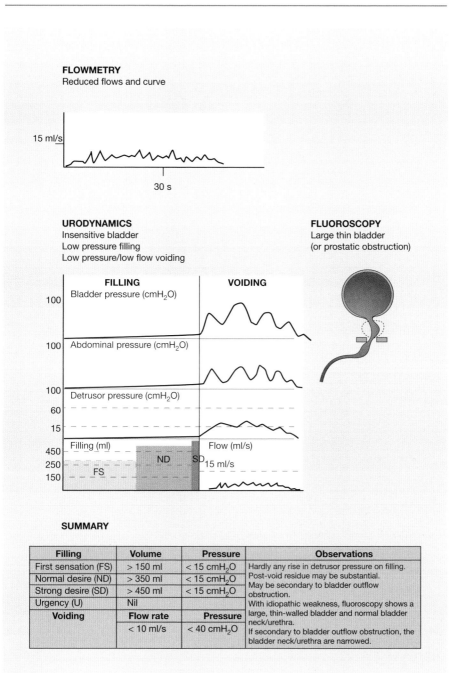

**FLOWMETRY**
Reduced flows and curve

15 ml/s

30 s

**URODYNAMICS**
Insensitive bladder
Low pressure filling
Low pressure/low flow voiding

**FLUOROSCOPY**
Large thin bladder
(or prostatic obstruction)

| FILLING | VOIDING |

Bladder pressure (cmH₂O) 100

Abdominal pressure (cmH₂O) 100

Detrusor pressure (cmH₂O) 100 / 60 / 15

Filling (ml) 450 / 250 / 150 — ND — SD — FS — Flow (ml/s) 15 ml/s

**SUMMARY**

| Filling | Volume | Pressure | Observations |
|---------|--------|----------|--------------|
| First sensation (FS) | > 150 ml | < 15 cmH₂O | Hardly any rise in detrusor pressure on filling. |
| Normal desire (ND) | > 350 ml | < 15 cmH₂O | Post-void residue may be substantial. |
| Strong desire (SD) | > 450 ml | < 15 cmH₂O | May be secondary to bladder outflow obstruction. |
| Urgency (U) | Nil | | With idiopathic weakness, fluoroscopy shows a |
| **Voiding** | **Flow rate** | **Pressure** | large, thin-walled bladder and normal bladder neck/urethra. |
| | < 10 ml/s | < 40 cmH₂O | If secondary to bladder outflow obstruction, the bladder neck/urethra are narrowed. |

Figure 8.8 Functional bladder abnormalities seen with detrusor weakness (e.g. idiopathic, as in this example, or secondary to long-standing outflow obstruction). The diagnostic abnormality is low voiding pressures (< 40 cmH₂O) with low flows (< 10 ml/s)

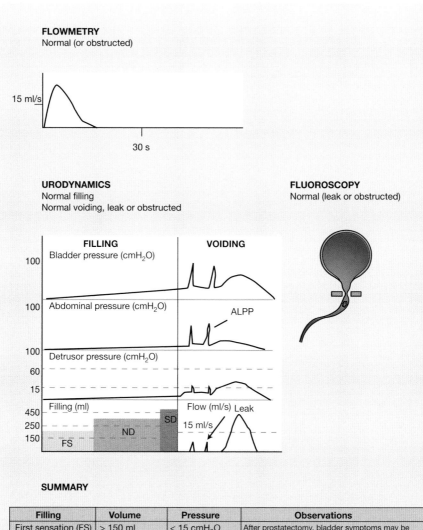

**FLOWMETRY**
Normal (or obstructed)

15 ml/s

30 s

**URODYNAMICS**
Normal filling
Normal voiding, leak or obstructed

**FLUOROSCOPY**
Normal (leak or obstructed)

FILLING     VOIDING

100 Bladder pressure (cmH₂O)

100 Abdominal pressure (cmH₂O)     ALPP

100 Detrusor pressure (cmH₂O)
60
15

450 Filling (ml)     Flow (ml/s) Leak
250    ND    SD    15 ml/s
150 FS

**SUMMARY**

| Filling | Volume | Pressure | Observations |
|---|---|---|---|
| First sensation (FS) | > 150 ml | < 15 cmH₂O | After prostatectomy, bladder symptoms may be due to anastomotic stricture with voiding figures consistent with bladder outflow obstruction, or the sphincter may be weak and features similar to genuine stress weakness (with leak pressure < 60 cmH₂O) are seen. Rarely, prostatectomy unmasks detrusor instability. |
| Normal desire (ND) | > 350 ml | < 15 cmH₂O | |
| Strong desire (SD) | > 450 ml | < 15 cmH₂O | |
| Urgency (U) | Nil | | |
| **Voiding** | **Flow rate** | **Pressure** | |
| | < 5 or > 25 ml/s | < or > 60 cmH₂O | |

Figure 8.9 Functional bladder abnormalities seen after prostatectomy. Voiding may be obstructed or not depending on whether the anastomosis is strictured; and fear of incontinence may manifest as reduced functional capacity and leakage may be demonstrated (thus appearance may be similar to Figures 8.5 and/or 8.6). ALPP, abdominal leak-point pressure

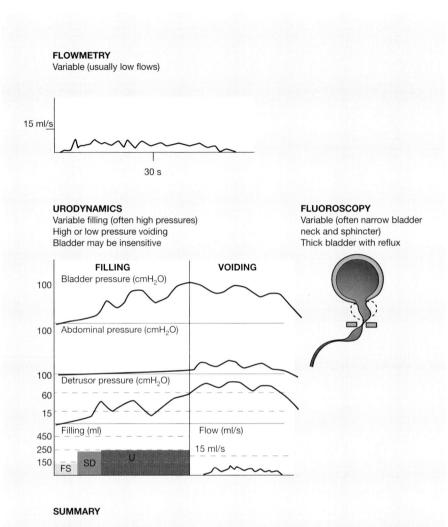

**FLOWMETRY**
Variable (usually low flows)

15 ml/s

30 s

**URODYNAMICS**
Variable filling (often high pressures)
High or low pressure voiding
Bladder may be insensitive

**FLUOROSCOPY**
Variable (often narrow bladder
neck and sphincter)
Thick bladder with reflux

FILLING    VOIDING

Bladder pressure (cmH$_2$O)
100

Abdominal pressure (cmH$_2$O)
100

Detrusor pressure (cmH$_2$O)
100
60
15

Filling (ml)         Flow (ml/s)
450
250                  15 ml/s
150
FS  SD    U

**SUMMARY**

| Filling | Volume | Pressure | Observations |
|---|---|---|---|
| First sensation (FS) | Nil, increased or decreased | < or > 15 cmH$_2$O | A variety of abnormalities may be seen |
| Normal desire (ND) | Nil, increased or decreased | < or > 15 cmH$_2$O | • reduced or absent bladder sensation |
| Strong desire (SD) | Nil, increased or decreased | < or > 15 cmH$_2$O | • detrusor acompliance |
| Urgency (U) | Nil | | • bladder neck or detrusor dyssynergia |
| **Voiding** | **Flow rate** | **Pressure** | • neurogenic detrusor overactivity |
| | Nil, > or < 15 ml/s | Low or increased | On fluoroscopy, bladder may be enlarged with a large residual, or thickened and shrunken with ureteric reflux |

Figure 8.10   Functional bladder abnormalities seen with a neuropathic bladder (this example shows detrusor overactivity as well as sphincter dyssynergia but other combinations are possible)

## Table 8.8 Complications of a neuropathic bladder

Ureteric reflux and upper tract dilatation (this is more common with poor compliance and if detrusor pressure is consistently $> 40 \, cmH_2O$)

Urinary tract infection

Urolithiasis

Autonomic dysreflexia*

*Lesions of the sympathetic outflow above T6. Bladder distension may result in paroxysmal hypertension, headache, sweating and bradycardia. This may require rapid treatment, because it can lead to subarachnoid haemorrhage.

# 9.   The Normal Urethra

- Anatomy
  Male
  Female
- Radiological Investigation of the Urethra
  Contrast Urethrography
      *Male*
      *Female*
  Ultrasound
      *Male*
      *Female*
- Other Imaging Modalities

## ANATOMY OF THE URETHRA

### The male urethra

The male urethra is divided into four parts; from proximal to distal these are the prostatic, membranous, bulbar and penile urethra (Figure 9.1). The prostatic urethra is the most proximal, commencing just below the bladder base and entirely enclosed within the prostate gland. It is also the widest, most distensible and

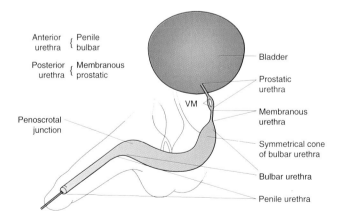

Figure 9.1   An illustration of the normal anterior urethra as seen on an ascending or anterior urethrogram (compare with Figure 9.2). VM, verumontanum

crescentic in outline. The mid-portion of the prostatic urethra is also called the verumontanum, where the paired ejaculatory ducts and the prostatic utricle are also located. The utricle is a blind-ending diverticulum that is a remnant of the paramesonephric ducts or the urogenital sinus, which in the female forms the reproductive tract.

The membranous portion commences as the urethra emerges from the prostatic apex and lies within the perineal membrane (also called the urogenital diaphragm or perineal body). It is the shortest portion (2 cm long) and is encircled by the external urethral sphincter. The levator ani muscles are its lateral relations, the rectum is posterior and the pubis is anterior. On emergence from the perineal membrane the anterior urethra commences. Terminologically, this is also split into the bulbar (that part in the bulb of the corpus spongiosum) and penile (within the pendulous part of the penis) urethra. The bulbo-urethral, Cowper's and paraurethral glands (of Littré) all drain into the bulbar urethra. The most distal part of the penile urethra widens in the navicular fossa but narrows at the urethral meatus.

The entire prostatic urethra is surrounded by variable amounts of circular and longitudinal smooth muscle fibres. Most proximally they merge with those around the bladder neck. Just below the bladder neck is the pre-prostatic sphincter which prevents retrograde ejaculation. Distally (within the perineal membrane) the muscles are separated by connective tissue from the striated muscle of the external sphincter, which is under voluntary control unlike the bladder neck.

## The female urethra

This is much shorter, at 3–4 cm long, and lies between the bladder neck and the external urethral meatus. It is less well supported by the pubo-urethral ligaments, which attach the urethra to the posterior part of the pubis symphysis, and the striated muscle of the external urethral sphincter.

## RADIOLOGICAL INVESTIGATION OF THE URETHRA

### Contrast urethrography in the male

The principal method for imaging of the male urethra is contrast urethrography. An ascending urethrogram is dedicated to the ascending urethra (i.e. the penile and bulbar urethra), while the descending urethrogram evaluates the posterior urethra (the prostatic and membranous urethra). The essential requisite for either study is adequate distension of the urethra. For the ascending urethrogram the anterior urethra is distended using either a Knudson's clamp or a Foley urethral catheter. The technique is described in Table 9.1. Once fully distended with con-

## Table 9.1    Male ascending urethrography (see also Figure 9.2)

**Equipment**

1.  Fluoroscopic facilities. Ideally digital imaging with fluoroscopic capture or store facilities. Subtraction imaging is not usually helpful

2.  Knudson's clamp or balloon Foley catheter (8–14 Fr) for distension of the urethra

**Method**

1.  The clamp or the balloon catheter is inserted using an aseptic technique. The use of any anaesthetic gel interferes with the efficacy of the seal and is best not used. The discomfort of the procedure can be managed by careful patient explanation and meticulous technique. In particular, the balloon of the Foley catheter (if used) should be distended only within the fossa naviculare until a seal is obtained, about 1–2 ml of fluid in the balloon is sufficient. Over-distension should be avoided, as this can traumatise the urethral mucosa

2.  The patient rotates his body to the right (about 45°). This movement straightens the urethra such that the full length will be visualised from the tip to the bladder neck. Further views are seldom necessary. The position of the external sphincter is better assessed on frontal views but the urethra is seen twisted on this view

3.  Moderately dilute iodinated contrast is used (200 g of iodine/ml) and 20–50 ml is necessary

4.  Contrast is injected, slowly to avoid intravasation, until the full length of the anterior urethra is seen well distended in profile

5.  To inject beyond the external sphincter, maintain a constant mild pressure till the sphincter relaxes and allows flow. It may take up to a minute for the sphincter to relax but this is preferable as forceful injection, as an attempt to bypass the sphincter, is seldom successful, is painful and may lead to contrast intravasation

6.  Images are taken when the urethra is well distended and contrast is seen to flow into the bladder. Further patient rotation may be necessary to visualise the true length and position of any stricture

7.  If micturition cystourethrography is necessary as well, the bladder is filled by retrograde injection or a catheter is inserted

**Modifications**

1.  Hypospadias, meatal stricture – insert a fine feeding catheter (6 Fr) through the narrowing. A seal can be created by tying a ribbon tape around the penis

2.  Bladder already catheterized, e.g. post-prostatectomy – a 6 Fr feeding tube can be teased adjacent to the catheter. Some gel may be helpful and a ribbon can be used to create a tight seal. The existing catheter may need to be advanced further so that its balloon does not obstruct the bladder neck

3.  Patient finds procedure too painful – this is rare but intravenous sedation should be considered

**Side-effects**

1.  Urinary tract infection: routine prophylactic antibiotics are not necessary (but see below)

2.  Urethral trauma: avoided by careful technique and gentle injection, antibiotics may be helpful

3.  Intravasation of contrast

4.  Contrast allergy, particularly with intravasation

trast medium, oblique images will show the full length of urethra from the navicular fossa to the external urethral sphincter and can be assessed for strictures and mucosal lesions. Contrast urethrography is currently indispensable for evaluation of trauma to the lower urinary tract. To study the descending or the posterior urethra, good distension can only be achieved by asking the man to micturate after the bladder has been filled with contrast media (Table 9.2). A micturating or

### Table 9.2 Micturating cystourethrography (see also Figures 9.3 and 9.4)

**Equipment**

1. Fluoroscopic facilities. Ideally, digital imaging with fluoroscopic capture or store facilities; a rotating C-arm is helpful

2. Bladder catheter

**Methods**

1. Patient is catheterised using an aseptic technique. Routine prophylactic antibiotics are unnecessary

2. Using a moderately dilute iodinated contrast medium the bladder is filled gently. Either use syringes to fill or gravity filling

3. Fill until well distended. Between 400 and 500 ml should be used if tolerated as the patient may not be able to micturate with smaller volumes

4. Intermittent fluoroscopy is used if bladder trauma is suspected and filling is stopped at the first sign of extravasation. The C-arm should be rotated so that the bladder is examined in multiple projections. This is also necessary to visualise the lower ureters for reflux

5. Spot films are taken in the anterior–posterior projection and both oblique projections once the bladder is full

6. The table is elevated. The patient stands on the platform at 30–45° rotation to see the urethra in profile during micturition. Men use a urinary bottle and women an appropriately designed funnel which is gripped by the thighs over the vaginal opening. Urinary flow rates can be measured at the same time (with corrections). Stress incontinence can be tested by asking the patient to cough during fluoroscopy. Pelvic floor descent can also be assessed

7. Micturition commences. Fluoroscopy is used and spot films are taken. The lower ureters should also be assessed

8. Post-micturition residue can be estimated

**Side-effects**

1. Urinary tract infection: over-zealous distension can lead to bacteraemia

2. Bladder trauma

3. Haematuria. This is usually mild, but antibiotics should be considered

descending urethrogram combined with an anterior urethrogram, will demonstrate the integrity or otherwise of the entire urethra and distended bladder. On first presentation with urethral disease a complete baseline (i.e. both an ascending and descending (Figures 9.2 and 9.3)) study is important, but for further follow-up only an ascending or descending study, or even ultrasound urethrography (below), are appropriate.

## Contrast urethrography in the female

The female urethra is much less prone to disease and there is no ideal imaging method. Ultrasound (either transvaginal or transrectal), micturating cystography and magnetic resonance imaging (MRI) can all help. The easiest, and the traditional, method is the micturating cystourethrogram, but as in the male, this

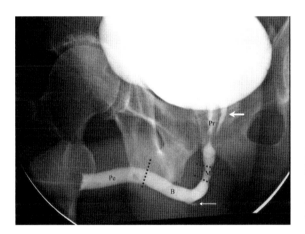

Figure 9.2 A normal ascending or anterior urethra. Pe, penile urethra; B, bulbar urethra; M, membranous urethra; Pr, prostatic urethra; thin arrow, Cowper's gland duct; thick arrow, persistent utricle

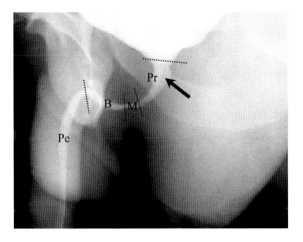

Figure 9.3 A normal descending urethrogram. Pe, penile urethra; B, bulbar urethra; M, membranous urethra; Pr, prostatic urethra; thick arrow, verumontanum

requires catheterisation and exposes the gonads to ionising radiation. The weakness of this study is that it is not sufficiently reliable to exclude a female urethral diverticulum (Figure 9.4) but in fact no imaging modality performs well in this area. The difficulty lies in achieving good urethral distension as, inevitably, inhibition on the part of the woman means that the bladder neck is not fully open and urinary flow is poor. This is made more difficult by the standing position necessary during this study. To overcome this limitation, a retrograde or ascending study would be necessary but this is very difficult in the woman because of the short urethra.

One method of retrograde female urethrography is the use of a double-balloon female urethral catheter. With this device both the bladder neck and the urethral orifice can be occluded by the two balloons, and contrast is injected into the short female urethra; better distension is achieved. Others have used just the rubber bung of the Knudson's device or a hysterosalpinogram catheter to achieve a satisfactory seal for good retrograde distension.

## Ultrasound of the urethra

Although in theory the urethra should be well visualised on ultrasound, in practice the examination is not straightforward, as, first, the posterior urethra in the male is partly covered by the interference from the pubic bones and, second, distension is required, which can be achieved in the male but of course not in the female. However, it does provide the opportunity to scrutinise the para-urethral soft tissues as well, unlike traditional contrast urethrography.

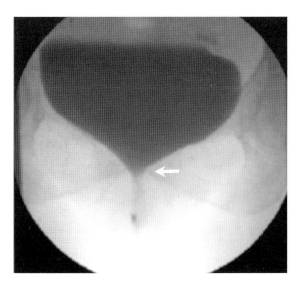

Figure 9.4 A micturating cystogram in a woman showing the normal female urethra

## Ultrasound urethrography in the male

In the male a superficial probe, such as a 7.5–12-MHz linear array probe, is used. The most convenient method is to distend the urethra using either a Knudson's clamp or a Foley catheter with the balloon distended in the navicular fossa. The urethra is distended using saline. An alternative distension agent is lignocaine gel or ultrasound gel, which can be made more transonic by initial agitation with air. An alternative would be the use of ultrasound contrast media but, unlike saline, all these other agents may obscure intraurethral bodies/calculi. In practical terms saline is the best agent. An alternative method is self-distension. After the urethral catheter has been inserted and the balloon has been inflated, the patient is asked to void against the balloon of the catheter, thereby self-distension of the entire urethra is produced. However, some men may be unable to void because of inhibition.

Once the urethra has been distended it is scanned in the transverse and longitudinal planes. Note is made of the smoothness of the urethral mucosal lining and discrepancies are noted and carefully examined. Both strictures and subtle wall irregularities of the anterior urethra are readily seen (Figure 9.5). The ability to visualise the stricture as well as the corresponding surrounding wall thickness or '(presumed) inflammatory' change is an advantage of this technique over contrast urethrography. Whether this additional information is of any clear advantage and helps in the selection of appropriate stricture therapy has not been proven. In theory the knowledge that a given stricture has significant associated abnormal, but unstrictured, mucosa may indicate that a longer length of urethroplasty is necessary and that surgery rather than optical urethrotomy is appropriate. However, controlled data on this aspect are lacking. The superiority of ultrasound over contrast urethrography is not yet proven.

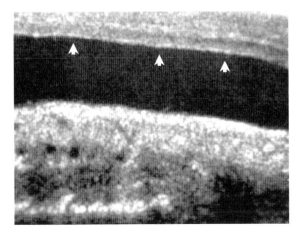

Figure 9.5 A normal ultrasound urethrogram showing a normal smooth urethral outline. This study is carried out after distension of the urethra with saline using a flat-array ultrasound probe (see text). Only the anterior urethra can be seen well by this method. Thus, unlike contrast urethrography, an ultrasound urethrogram is not a global study of the urethra

The urethra can be scanned easily up to the membranous urethra using longitudinal scanning, but the posterior urethra will be insufficiently visualised. To visualise better the posterior urethra transperineal scanning with a 3.5–5-MHz curved array probe can be used, or a transrectal probe (Figure 9.6) can be used. Distension of the posterior urethra is only well achieved by asking the man to void. Overall posterior ultrasound urethrography is much less reliable than micturating or descending contrast urethrography.

To summarise, ultrasound urethrography is a suitable technique for visualising the male anterior urethra, being as good as ascending contrast urethrography in published series. Whether it is better remains to be proven. It, of course, has the advantage of avoiding ionising radiation, an important consideration as most urethral stricture disease occurs in the young and the testes are in direct line of the beam with contrast urethrography. Its disadvantages are that it is possibly more cumbersome, particularly if the self-voiding technique is used for distension, global studies of the urethra (i.e. both the anterior and posterior urethra) are less easily obtained (and possibly the posterior urethral views are less reliable) and, finally, it is not suitable for the assessment of early urethral trauma. As yet, ultrasound urethrography cannot replace contrast urethrography but should be seriously considered as a follow-up option in the man with known anterior urethral stricture.

## Ultrasound urethrography in the female

This is much less convenient than the comparable study, that is micturating cystourethrography, as the transrectal or transvaginal route is necessary during the

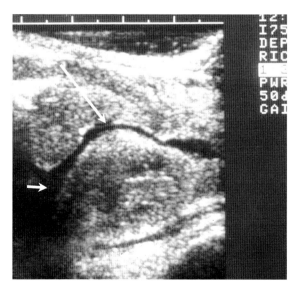

Figure 9.6 This view is an ultrasound study of the posterior urethra (short arrow is the bladder neck, long arrow is the prostatic urethra). To study the posterior urethra by ultrasound, scanning needs to be performed via the transperineal or transrectal route

**Table 9.3  Magnetic resonance imaging of the urethra**

**Pre-procedure**
Pelvic surface coil is used
In the male the penis is taped in the midline to the anterior abdominal wall

Urethral distension is achieved in the male (the balloon of the catheter is inflated in the fossa naviculare and the urethra is distended with saline injection)

**Procedure**
Small field of view
Thin section (3–5 mm) acquisitions
Male and female patients
- T1 and T2 axial
- T1 and T2 sagittal

Other sequences useful
- post-contrast T1 (axial and sagittal)
- post-cavernosal distension (using prostaglandin injection)

voiding phase. Non-voiding studies can be carried out using transperineal (or labial) curved array ultrasonography but evaluation is difficult. One area, however, where ultrasound may be of particular value is in the evaluation for a urethral diverticulum. This abnormality is notoriously difficult to exclude, but sometimes the diverticulum can be easily seen on ultrasound at rest and any contained calculus will be seen.

## OTHER IMAGING MODALITIES

Of the other imaging modalities MRI has the potential to provide significant additional information compared to contrast or ultrasound urethrography but it has not been fully exploited. This is because distension is difficult to achieve and maintain within the small bore of the MRI machine. The technical details are given in Table 9.3. Currently, it is used mainly for the staging of urethral cancers.

# 10. CONGENITAL ANOMALIES OF THE URETHRA

- POSTERIOR URETHRAL VALVES
- URETHRAL DUPLICATION
- CONGENITAL MEATAL OR URETHRAL STENOSIS
- HYPOSPADIAS
- MEGALOURETHRA
- ANTERIOR URETHRAL DIVERTICULUM
- COWPER'S DUCT CYST OR SYRINGOCOELE

## POSTERIOR URETHRAL VALVES

Although usually diagnosed in childhood, posterior urethral valves can occasionally present in adult life. The cause is unknown and they may be classified anatomically (types 1–3) or according to the degree of upper tract dilatation (mild, moderate, or severe). Diagnosis rests on the findings of a dilated posterior urethra on micturating cystourethrography (ureteric reflux may also be seen in about 50% of cases). The valve is seen as a filling defect just above the point of transition between a dilated posterior urethra and a normal or attenuated anterior urethra (Figure 10.1). Oblique views are important and the filling catheter should be removed. Sonography can also be used to diagnose valves, either by the transabdominal or transperineal route. In the adult transrectal ultrasound can also be used. However, ascending urethrography will not always show the valve as it is flattened by the jet of contrast.

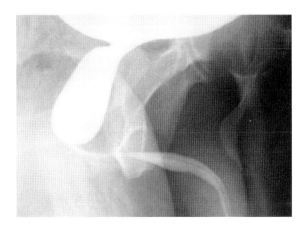

Figure 10.1 A micturating cystogram showing a posterior urethral valve resulting in outflow obstruction

## URETHRAL DUPLICATION

This is a rare anomaly and may be partial or complete. A blind, duplicated urethra may also occur (Figure 10.2) and rarely there may also be a duplicated bladder. The structures are best demonstrated by thorough ascending and descending urethrography; this may require catheterisation of both urethras.

## CONGENITAL MEATAL OR URETHRAL STENOSIS

The meatus may be pinpoint in calibre from birth, but this anomaly is much less common than acquired meatal stenosis. Meatal stenosis may be associated with hypospadias but it may also occur as a complication of circumcision. If radiological evaluation is required, e.g. to assess the length of the stenosis and to exclude any further unsuspected urethral strictures, then ascending urethrography can best be carried out using a 6-Fr feeding catheter. This is manipulated past the narrowed meatus and good distended views are possible, although further occlusion can be achieved by pinching the bulb of the penis around the feeding catheter. A micturating study is also useful, as the full length of the urethra will be demonstrated (Figure 10.3). Congenital urethral stenosis is also uncommon and occurs at the junction of the posterior and anterior urethras. Its cause is not known.

## HYPOSPADIAS

In this condition the urethral meatus opens onto the ventral aspect of the penis or the perineum and there may also be a ventral curvature. Other associations are

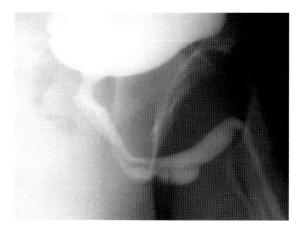

Figure 10.2 A partly duplicated anterior urethra

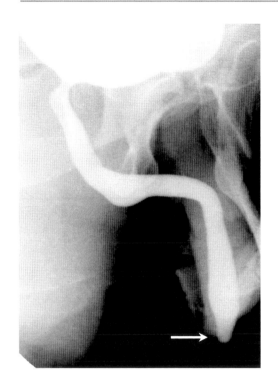

Figure 10.3 A micturating cystogram demonstrating meatal stenosis (arrow)

undescended testicles, inguinal hernia, urinary tract anomalies (duplication, pelvic-ureteric junction obstruction), imperforate anus and Müllerian duct remnants. There may be an associated meatal stenosis as explained above.

## MEGALOURETHRA AND ANTERIOR URETHRAL DIVERTICULUM

In this curious condition both the urethra and the corpus spongiosum are maldeveloped. The urethra is massively dilated and may involve the whole anterior urethra, because the entire spongiosum is maldeveloped, or may be localized secondary to a focal defect in the spongiosum. The more severe variety is less common and usually associated with other severe maldevelopments. The less common localized megalourethra (Figure 10.4) (sometimes called the scaphoid megalourethra) may also present with upper urinary tract anomalies and prune belly syndrome. The scaphoid megalourethra is also called anterior urethral diverticulum. In the existing literature it is not clear whether these two conditions are truly separate entities, however, it is said that the diverticulum may be associated with a lip-like 'anterior urethral valve' which may be obstructive during voiding studies.

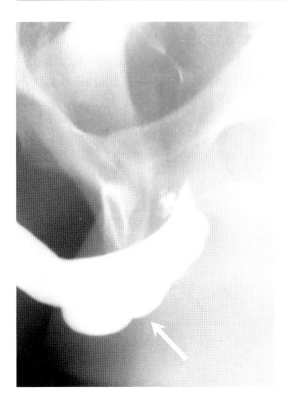

Figure 10.4 Partial megalo-urethra of the bulbar urethra (arrow)

## COWPER'S DUCT CYST OR SYRINGOCOELE

The Cowper's ducts are periurethral glands and are accessory sex glands that help to lubricate the semen. They are located in the membranous or the bulbar urethra and their ducts open as separate units or singly into the proximal bulbar urethra. The commonest anomaly is the Cowper's duct cyst, which is sometimes termed a syringocoele. It is a retention cyst and is believed to be a congenital abnormality. It usually presents in childhood, however, the occasional case may be first encountered during adulthood (Figure 10.5). It is postulated that the adult Cowper's duct cyst is the result of postinflammatory stricturing of the duct, the result of either infection or instrumentation. The underlying fault is obstruction of the duct of the Cowper's gland, which results in cystic dilatation. It may be an incidental finding, or it may present with urinary infections, obstructed voiding, post-micturition dribbling or lower urinary tract symptoms (frequency, urgency).

Characteristically it is seen as a smooth indentation of the ventral surface of the anterior urethra on contrast urethrography, but may be recognised on ultrasound or magnetic resonance imaging as a thin-walled cystic structure (Figure 10.5).

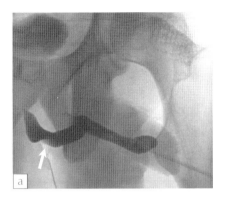

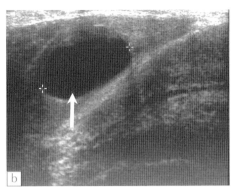

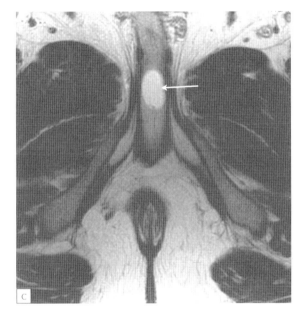

Figure 10.5 Images demonstrating the urethrographic (indentation of the ventral surface of the anterior urethra (a)), sonographic (b) and T2 weighted magnetic resonance imaging (c) appearances of a Cowper's duct cyst (arrows)

# 11. Intraluminal Abnormalities and Filling Defects of the Urethra

- Calculi
- Foreign Bodies
- Hair Balls
- Urethral Polyp

Intraluminal or mucosal abnormalities of the urethra are best appreciated during well-distended contrast or ultrasound urethrography. Overall they are uncommon findings compared to urethral strictures or traumatic abnormalities, but some of these abnormalities, in particular calculi, may occur in common with stricture disease. Table 11.1 lists the causes of filling defects seen on urethrography.

## CALCULI

Stones can form *in situ* within the urethra or migrate down from the upper urinary tract or bladder. Passage of stones is usually only a temporary event as the stone is evacuated naturally, unless there is a structural abnormality present, such as a stricture or a diverticulum, that prevents stone expulsion. 'Primary' urethral calculi usually form as a result of an underlying urethral abnormality. Examples are stricture, diverticulum, prior urethroplasty with an area of redundancy, or secondary diverticulum. Occasionally after urethroplasty using a flap of hair-bearing skin, hair follicles overgrow into a hair ball which may calcify.

Secondary calculi migrate down from the bladder, are more common and may present acutely with obstruction. In comparison, primary calculi present with

| Table 11.1   Filling defects in the urethra | |
|---|---|
| Calculi | Congenital urethral polyp |
| Foreign body | Acquired urethral polyp |
| Bezoar or hair ball | Ureterocoele |
| Blood clot | Urethritis cystica |
| Posterior urethral valve | Neoplasm |

chronic symptoms, such as urethral bleeding or infections. Both types may be seen on a precontrast radiograph but they are usually faintly opaque and may be missed. On ascending urethrography they may be easily overlooked or mistaken for air bubbles because they are small and poorly opaque (Figure 11.1). All urethrograms that show a diverticulum or stricture should be carefully evaluated for missed calculi. Stones are much more readily appreciated on ultrasound urethrography as a typical shadow-casting, highly reflectile object.

## FOREIGN BODIES

A plethora of intraurethral (and intravesical) foreign bodies have been described in the literature. They are almost all self-inserted and beyond marvelling at the imaginative variety of objects chosen, there is little more to say on this subject. Most are radio-opaque and obvious on plain radiographs (Figures 11.2 and 11.3). Small objects, however, may have been forgotten and may be encountered on later urethrography either as a filling defect or as a formed calculus.

## HAIR BALLS

These are much less commonly seen now. They first came to general notice after a vogue for urethroplasty using myofascial flaps for urethral surgery and reconstruction. The retained hair follicles of the epidermis after shedding built up into a foreign body that may eventually have calcified.

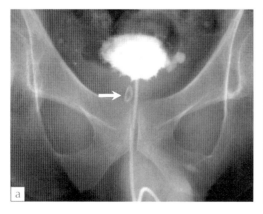 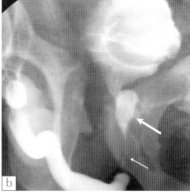

Figure 11.1   (a) Two urethrographic images showing urethral calculi (thick arrow); (b) also shows a membranous stricture post-trauma (thin arrow)

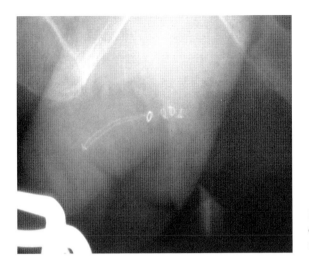

Figure 11.2 Foreign bodies (wire material) in the anterior urethra

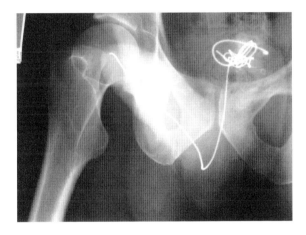

Figure 11.3 Another example of foreign bodies (wire material) in the anterior urethra and bladder

## POLYPS OF THE MALE URETHRA

These are usually congenital polyps and are most commonly seen in the posterior urethra. Polyps of the anterior urethra are much less common. At both sites they are histologically benign and covered with transitional epithelium, occasionally with areas of squamous metaplasia. They usually present in childhood with obstructive symptoms because the polyp is usually on a long stalk and acts as a ball-valve, obstructing urine flow during micturition. The obstruction may be severe and prolonged such that there may be associated features of long-standing, high-pressure voiding with bladder trabeculation or retention, hydroureter and hydronephrosis.

The diagnosis is usually made on ascending or descending urethrography. The stalk of the polyp may be long and the polyp may protrude into the bladder and be seen as an intravesical filling defect. This can mimic a ureterocoele on contrast studies but is easily differentiated on ultrasound because a polyp is seen to be a solid structure unlike the transonic, cystic appearance of a ureterocoele.

# 12. Intrinsic Abnormalities of the Urethral Wall

- Urethritis
- Urethral Strictures
- Female Urethral Diverticulum
- Male Urethral Diverticulum

## URETHRITIS

Inflammation of the urethral mucosa is very common but most cases are easily treated and do not come to radiological attention. The three main causes are uncomplicated gonococcal urethritis, *Chlamydia trachomatis* infection and other non-specific urethritis, caused by *Ureaplasma urealyticum, Trichomonas vaginalis* and, rarely, herpes simplex virus. In the acute stage, if imaging is carried out, a subtle irregularity is seen related to the anterior urethra. More chronic cases result in urethral strictures.

## URETHRAL STRICTURES

The majority of urethral strictures occur in the anterior male urethra. Stricture of the female urethra is uncommon and more usually the result of mobility and kinking of the urethra rather than as a result of fibrosis. This is an example of a 'functional' stricture of the urethra. Table 12.1 lists the various other causes of urethral strictures encountered in current practice.

Irrespective of the cause of the urethral stricture, on imaging certain general rules apply, all of which are directed at providing appropriate information to guide the management of the patient rather than to diagnose specifically the underlying cause. The cause may always remain obscure in a given patient. The most important information for guiding treatment is accurately to locate the site of the stricture, the length of the stricture (Figures 12.1 and 12.2) and the proximity of the stricture to the external urethral sphincter. A one-stage imaging pathway that can provide all this information is important.

Conventionally, an ascending and descending cystourethrogram is chosen and is ideally suited for this purpose. The exact location and length of the stricture is seen, particularly on oblique views (Figures 12.2 and 12.3). A thickened trabecu-

## Table 12.1 Causes of urethral strictures encountered in current practice

**Congenital**
Meatal stenosis (with hypospadias)
Prune belly syndrome

**Post-inflammatory**
Gonorrhoea
*Chlamydia* and non-specific urethritis
Tuberculosis
Schistosomiasis
*Mycoplasma*

**Post-traumatic**
Pelvic fractures
(straddle injury of the bulbar urethra)

**Iatrogenic**
Catheters
Cystoscopy

**Postoperative**
Post-urethroplasty
Post-prostatectomy

**'Functional'**
Benign prostatic hyperplasia
Detrusor sphincter dyssynergia
Bladder neck dyssynergia

**Tumour**
Squamous cell carcinoma
Transitional cell carcinoma

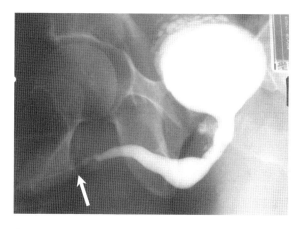

Figure 12.1 Long stricture of the penile urethra, causing bladder wall thickening and trabeculation

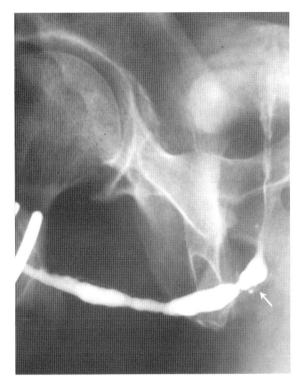

Figure 12.2 Post-inflammatory, multiple strictures of the anterior urethra, amounting to pan-urethritis of the anterior urethra. Filling of the Cowper's duct is also seen (arrow)

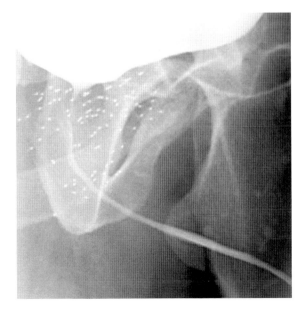

Figure 12.3 Post-radiation, severe narrowing of the posterior urethra. Radio-opaque radiation 'seeds' are also seen

lated bladder is an indirect indication of high-pressure voiding and ureteral reflux with hydronephrosis may be seen.

Finally any incomplete bladder emptying with a post-void residue is seen on the micturition studies. Further important information is the presence of urethral diverticula, false passages, stones (Figure 11.1) and abscesses. Analysis of the outline of the non-strictured urethra around the narrowing will demonstrate if the extent of diseased mucosa is longer than suspected from the narrowed area alone. This is better visualised on ultrasound urethrography, but this does not provide a global study. However, the value of diagnosing such ultrasonographically defined unhealthy mucosa (Figure 12.4) has not been proven.

The purpose of this information is to guide the surgeon in choosing a suitable course of management. Unfortunately, at the time of writing there is no clear consensus as to the best treatment for urethral strictures. In general terms, anterior urethral strictures < 1 cm in length with healthy surrounding mucosa are treated by optical urethrotomy (Figures 12.4a and 12.5). Longer strictures are treated by urethroplasty (Figure 12.4b), best carried out as a bucccal mucosa onlay graft, and the treatment of diffuse stricture disease of the penile urethra (Figure 12.2) remains problematic and is managed by either repeated dilatation or total urethroplasty.

## FEMALE URETHRAL DIVERTICULUM

This rare condition (incidence ranges from 0.6 to 3%, but even this is likely to be an overestimation) is characterized by late diagnosis. The peak age of diagnosis is

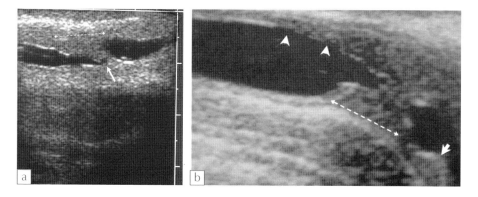

Figure 12.4 (a) An ultrasound urethrogram showing a discrete stricture in the anterior urethra (arrow). (b) An ultrasound urethrogram showing a stricture in the anterior urethra (hatched arrow) but the abnormal mucosa is more extensive than estimated by just measurement of the length of the stricture (the arrowheads indicate the extent of the abnormal urethral mucosa)

the mid-forties and the symptoms are usually non-specific – classically, dribbling after micturition, dysuria and dyspareunia. Some cases are asymptomatic, but others are associated with infection, bladder outlet obstruction, incontinence, calculi (Figure 12.6) and, rarely, malignancy. The cancer is usually adenocarcinoma.

Radiological diagnosis is difficult as well and a variety of modalities have been used (Figures 12.6 and 12.7). Micturating cystourethrogram is said to be positive

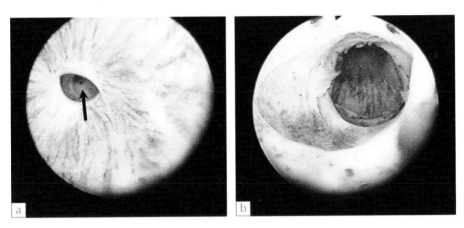

Figure 12.5   Endoscopic views of a stricture (arrow) in the anterior urethra, before (a) and after (b) optical urethrotomy. (Figure courtesy of Mr K. Anson)

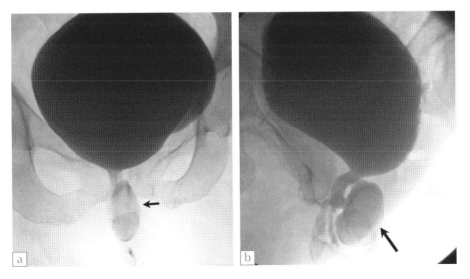

Figure 12.6   Frontal (a) and oblique (b) views of a female urethral diverticulum demonstrated on micturating cystography. There is a calculus (arrow) in the diverticulum (image courtesy of Dr C. Allen)

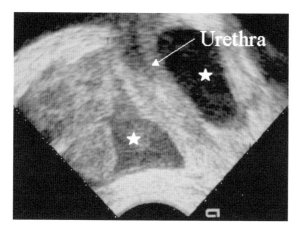

Figure 12.7 A transrectal ultrasound image showing a bilobed (stars) female urethral diverticulum. There is echogenic material seen in the posterior diverticulum (image courtesy of Dr C. Allen)

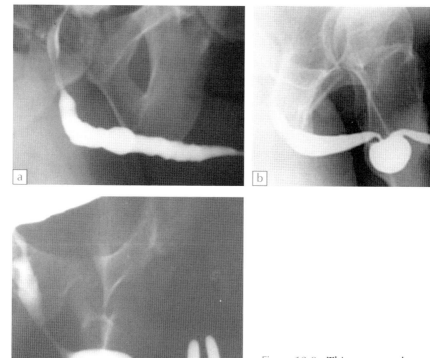

Figure 12.8 This montage shows three examples of urethral diverticula in men. (a) Shows a post-inflammatory diverticulum, (b) is postoperative and (c) occurred after urethral trauma

in up to 95% of cases, while urethrography with a double-balloon catheter will identify around 90% of diverticula. In others, transvaginal or transrectal ultrasonography (Figure 12.7) has successfully demonstrated the abnormality and, more recently, magnetic resonance imaging has been evaluated. In one study the sensitivities of micturating cystourethrography, double-balloon urethrography and transvaginal ultrasonography were 77%, 86% and 100%, respectively; and in a separate study, magnetic resonance imaging showed a diverticulum in three women with false-negative results on double-balloon urethrography. Thus, it seems in modern clinical practice women with a clinical suspicion of diverticulum should be investigated with transvaginal/transrectal ultrasonography and magnetic resonance imaging. If these are unhelpful, a micturition cystogram should be carried out and double balloon urethrography should be reserved for rare cases.

## MALE URETHRAL DIVERTICULUM

These are acquired mainly after injury, infection or long-term urethral catheterisation; and are typically in the ventral surface at the penoscrotal junction or in the bulbar urethra (Figure 12.8). Clinical presentation is with urinary tract infection, post-void dribbling, or poor urinary stream. Ascending urethrogram or ultrasound urethrogram will demonstrate the abnormality without difficulty.

# 13. Lower Urinary Tract Trauma

- Bladder Trauma
  Causes
  Classification
- Urethral Trauma
  Causes
  Classification
  Investigation
  Male
  Female

Trauma of the lower urinary tract is usually the result of pelvic injury. At the time of presentation lower urinary tract trauma may be suspected if there is urethral bleeding or urinary retention. If so, lower tract imaging should be carried out to exclude any injury prior to catheter insertion. Bladder and urethral injuries are dealt with here under separate subsections but they can occur together.

## BLADDER TRAUMA

With its location deep within the pelvis the bladder is generally protected from external trauma. When injured the causes are pelvic fracture, direct blow to a distended bladder, direct penetrating trauma or an iatrogenic accident, usually inadvertent operative injury (Table 13.1). Prompt diagnosis improves outcomes.

Blunt injury is the commonest cause and occurs in 1.6% of blunt abdominal trauma cases. The majority are associated with pelvic fractures and about 6% of all pelvic fractures are associated with some bladder trauma. Often bladder injury is combined with urethral trauma – this is seen in about 10–20% of cases with bladder injury.

The investigation of choice is cystography, but it is important to fill the bladder sufficiently to 'stress' the bladder. A volume of 400 ml should be instilled under low pressure or gravity infusion under intermittent fluoroscopy, and a post-drainage film should be obtained to avoid missing subtle posterior leaks at the base of the bladder. A similar study can be carried out under computerised tomography (CT). 'CT cystography' is as accurate as traditional cystography but again adequate bladder distension should be ensured.

| Table 13.1 Causes of bladder trauma |
| --- |

Blunt injury
- wall contusion

Pelvic fracture
- intraperitoneal bladder rupture
- extraperitoneal bladder rupture

Penetrating injury

Iatrogenic injury
- pelvic surgery (obstetric/gynaecological)
- pelvic fracture repair
- during aorto-iliac surgery
- during bladder catheterisation (suprapubic)

Mild injury may only result in bladder wall contusion, and the integrity of the wall is maintained. Extravasation of contrast does not occur. The bladder outline is distorted but this may be overlooked on cystography if the distortion is small or affects the anterior wall. Intraperitoneal bladder rupture occurs in about 40% of cases (Figure 13.1) and is the result of a sudden rise in intravesical pressure after a direct blow to the bladder. The tear is usually at the dome. On cystography, contrast will outline the intraperitoneal structures and fill the paracolic gutters.

Extraperitoneal rupture is almost always due to pelvic fracture (Figure 13.2). The bladder is seared anteriorly at the base because of disruption of the bony pelvic ring. On cystography the bladder may be seen to have assumed a teardrop or pear shape, because it is compressed by haematoma of the pelvic side walls (Figure 7.1). Contrast will leak from the base of the bladder and track along the side walls. Extensive injury may result in contrast extravasation into the anterior abdominal wall, or to the thigh or scrotum via the obturator and inguinal foramina, respectively. Rarely, both an extra- and an intraperitoneal rupture may occur.

Penetrating injury may be the result of either a knife or a gunshot. Marked haematuria is seen and cystography will confirm the tear/disruption. Iatrogenic injuries occur most frequently during obstetric or gynaecological procedures. Laparoscopic procedures increase the risk of this injury. The majority are recognised at the time of injury and are immediately corrected. If not, diagnosis is delayed and best recognised by cystography.

## INJURY OF THE MALE URETHRA

Injury to the urethra also most commonly occurs after pelvic trauma and in the younger male (merely because major pelvic trauma is more common in this age

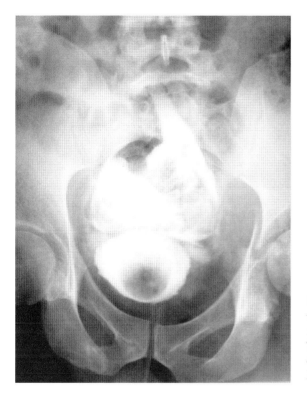

Figure 13.1 A cystographic view of intraperitoneal bladder rupture after pelvic trauma. This may be overlooked if the contrast rapidly dilutes into a large intraperitoneal urinoma

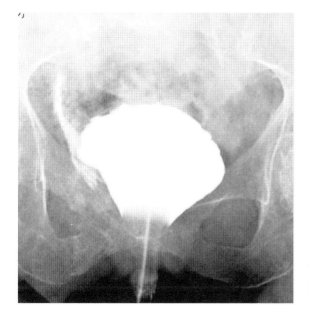

Figure 13.2 A cystographic view demonstrating extraperitoneal bladder leak after pelvic trauma

group). The injuries are often not life threatening and do not result in any major systemic upset, unlike major bladder trauma. The long-term consequences may be urethral stricture, incontinence, or impotence, depending on whether the anterior urethra is involved, the external sphincter is damaged, or if there is associated injury to the neurovascular bundles. Table 13.2 lists the type and site of injuries and causes other than blunt pelvic trauma.

Anterior urethral injuries are less common (about 33%) as the anterior urethra is a relatively mobile structure. They are usually the result of direct trauma to the relatively exposed penile and bulbar urethra (Figure 13.3). The corpora spongiosum and the bulbar urethra are compressed against the pubic symphysis disrupting the urethra. If the Buck fascia remains intact the bruising is limited to the space between the fascia and the tunica albuginea. However, if the Buck fascia is also disrupted the blood, and contrast media, extravasates more widely up to the scrotum, perineum, or anterior abdominal wall, and extensive soft-tissue bruising is seen. Posterior urethral injury implies major life-threatening pelvic fractures. The posterior urethra is within the bony pelvis and generally protected from trauma unless the pelvic ring is disrupted. The mechanism involves shearing of the

---

**Table 13.2   Urethral injuries**

**Anterior urethra**

Blunt trauma
• 	falls astride/perineal kicks

Penetrating trauma
• 	gunshot/knife wounds

Sexual excess
• 	penile fractures

Iatrogenic injuries
• 	urethral catheters
• 	urethroscopy
• 	penile surgery

**Posterior urethra**

Penetrating injuries
• 	gunshot/knife wounds

Pelvic fractures
• 	road traffic accidents

Iatrogenic injuries
• 	endoscopic surgery, transurethral resection of the prostate

urethra at the prostatic apex and the puboprostatic ligaments; with the prostate being driven cephalad. Between 3 and 25% of pelvic fractures are associated with urethral injuries and in 10–20% there may be an associated bladder injury.

It is important to locate the site of injury precisely as it has some bearing on the chosen treatment. Table 13.3 describes the classification system currently used for urethral trauma.

## Investigation of suspected urethral trauma

If urethral injury is suspected (blood at the meatus, gross haematuria, inability to void, or a high prostate on per-rectal examination) then urethral investigations are necessary prior to the insertion of a per-urethral catheter. Blind insertion may convert a partial injury into a complete tear. The standard technique is retrograde or ascending urethrography. Properly conducted, this can classify the injury accordingly (Table 13.3 and Figures 13.3–13.6). If the result is non-diagnostic then a suprapubic catheter is inserted and urethral studies are repeated at a later date.

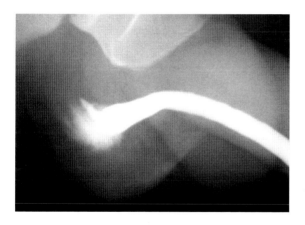

Figure 13.3 An ascending urethrogram showing complete pure anterior urethral injury (type 5 injury)

| Table 13.3 | Classification of urethral trauma |
| --- | --- |
| Class | Site of injury |
| 1 | Posterior urethra stretched but integrity is maintained |
| 2 | Tear of the membranous urethra, above the urogenital diaphragm |
| 3 | Partial or complete tear of both anterior and posterior urethra, with disruption of the urogenital diaphragm |
| 4 | Bladder injury extending into the urethra |
| 4a | Injury of the bladder base, with periurethral extravasation |
| 5 | Partial or complete pure anterior urethral injury |

However, a contrast urethrogram provides no information regarding the surrounding soft-tissue injuries; and spasm at the external sphincter may prevent visualisation of the posterior urethra and bladder.

Most patients with major pelvic trauma will also be subjected to CT and some signs have been described that may help to classify the level of urethral trauma from these CT data. A distance between the prostatic apex and the urogenital diaphragm of > 2 mm is seen with type 1 injury. Types 2 and 3 may be distinguished by the contrast extravasation above and below the urogenital diaphragm, respectively. However, the experience with CT is still not sufficient and it cannot replace contrast urethrography. Magnetic resonance imaging (MRI) is seldom carried out in the acute phase, although it has the potential to delineate the sites of injury and the surrounding tissues well. Ultrasound urethrography is not yet sufficiently well evaluated to be recommended.

The above relates to imaging in the acute situation. For later imaging prior to delayed urethral reconstruction, contrast urethrography is again the investigation

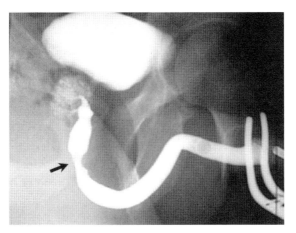

Figure 13.4 An ascending urethrogram showing a tear of the prostatic urethra above the urogenital diaphragm with extravasation (type 2 injury). The arrow indicates the level of the urogenital diaphragm

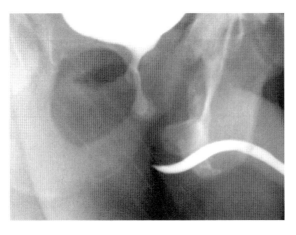

Figure 13.5 A simultaneous ascending and descending study carried out to demonstrate the length of the 'defect' prior to surgical reconstruction. A type 2 injury

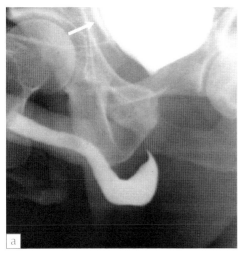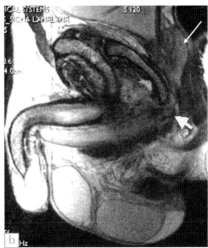

Figure 13.6 A simultaneous ascending and descending contrast study (a) with magnetic resonance imaging (MRI) correlation (b). MRI can be potentially more informative than the contrast study, as it also demonstrates the surrounding structures. In (a) the arrow points to the extraperitoneal leak from the bladder base, but the MRI shows that injury extends into the urethra (thick arrow in (b) points to the disrupted prostatic urethra, thin arrow indicates the prostate gland) confirming that this is a type 4 injury. However, to date, MRI has not been proven to be superior to contrast urethrography, and is a difficult study to carry out immediately after trauma

of choice. If there is discontinuity of the urethra then simultaneous ascending and descending studies (the latter carried out using a suprapubic catheter to fill the bladder) or the so-called 'up and downogram' will show the length of the defect to best advantage (Figure 13.5). MRI has also been used for delayed evaluation of urethral trauma and can show the length of the defect just as accurately, as well as showing the status of the surrounding tissues (Figure 13.6).

## INJURY OF THE FEMALE URETHRA

Because of its shorter length, higher elasticity and the absence of any substantial ligamentous attachments to the pubic bones, the female urethra is rarely injured during blunt trauma, although there is evidence to suggest underdiagnosis. When it occurs the injuries are severe and they often have associated rectal and vaginal injuries. Diagnosis is difficult and some have suggested that vaginoscopy and urethroscopy can be helpful. Other more common causes of injury to the female urethra are instrumentation, vaginal surgery and obstetric complications.

# 14. Neoplasms of the Urethra

- Benign Tumours
- Urethral Carcinoma
- Staging of Urethral Carcinoma

These may be encountered as filling defects on urethrography or strictures, but whether benign or malignant, both are rare findings. Table 14.1 lists the various types of urethral tumours that may be seen.

## BENIGN TUMOURS

The commonest benign tumour of the anterior or posterior urethra is the urethral polyp, as discussed in Chapter 11. Sometimes also called the fibrous urethral polyp, it presents with obstructive symptoms and is seen as a smooth, mobile, fill-

| Table 14.1   Tumours of urethra |
| --- |
| **Benign** |
| Benign prostatic epithelial polyp |
| Haemangioma |
| Leiomyoma |
| **Malignant** |
| Squamous cell carcinoma |
| Transitional cell carcinoma |
| Adenocarcinoma |
| Sarcoma |
| Melanoma |
| Metastatic <br> • prostate <br> • bladder <br> • testis <br> • colon <br> • kidney |

ing defect. Of the others, rare cases of haemangioma or leiomyoma have been described, with no particular distinguishing features but magnetic resonance imaging (MRI) has the potential to be diagnostically discriminating in these situations.

## URETHRAL CARCINOMA

Fewer than 1% of all urinary tract cancers occur within the urethra, however, they are more common in males (by a ratio of 7 : 3) with a peak age of onset in the seventh decade. Nearly 80% are squamous cell carcinoma, some 15% are of transitional cell origin and the rest are adenocarcinoma. In the male the commonest site is the anterior urethra, with most occurring in the bulbar urethra (60% in the bulbo-membranous urethra, 30% in the penile urethra and 10% within the prostatic urethra). Of the recognised risk factors, there may be a history of venereal disease in one-third of cases, a history of urethral stricture in a further one-third of cases and 5–7% may report a history of urethral trauma. Adenocarcinomas originate in the glands of Littré or Cowper's gland.

Presentation may be with obstructive symptoms, a palpable mass, a periurethral abscess or fistula. Diagnosis is often delayed and 50% of patients have metastatic disease at presentation. On urethrography, a long, narrow, irregular stricture is seen (Figures 14.1 and 14.2). A filling defect or mass lesion is a less common appearance; this is more often seen with benign lesions such as a polyp. Sometimes urethral carcinoma presents as a change in appearance of a known or long-standing urethral stricture; or as a new stricture occurrence after previous urethroplasty.

In women 60% of urethral carcinoma are squamous cell urethral carcinoma, 20% are transitional cell carcinoma with adenocarcinomas and undifferentiated

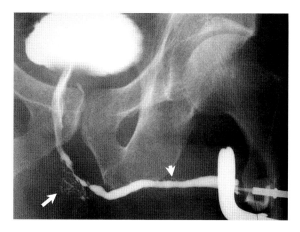

Figure 14.1 Ascending urethrogram demonstrating irregularity and extravasation (arrow) from the bulbar urethra, as well as further bulbar urethral strictures. This was a urethral carcinoma that had developed in a patient with chronic postinflammatory urethral strictures. The arrowhead indicates periurethral glands

tumours comprising the remaining 20%. They may occur within a female urethral diverticulum. Most squamous cell tumours occur in the distal third of the urethra, whilst the other cell types are more common in the proximal urethra. Presentation is usually with a bleeding urethral mass, best assessed with cross-sectional imaging, particularly MRI. Radiological staging of both male and female urethral cancers is best performed by MRI as well (Figure 14.3). The tumour–node–metastasis (TNM) staging system is given in Table 14.2.

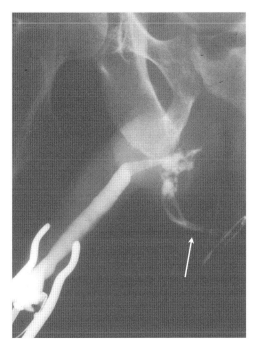

Figure 14.2 Ascending urethrogram demonstrating a squamous cell carcinoma of the bulbar urethra with a fistula (arrow)

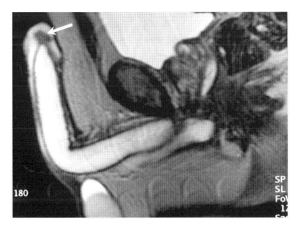

Figure 14.3 T2-weighted magnetic resonance imaging (MRI) scan of the penis demonstrating a carcinoma at the tip involving the glans (arrow). This was a penile cancer, but MRI is the modality of choice for staging of urethral cancers

## Table 14.2  TNM classification of urethral carcinoma

**T – Primary tumour**

TX – primary tumour cannot be assessed

T0 – no evidence of primary tumour

Ta – non-invasive papillary, polypoid, or verrucous carcinoma

Tis – carcinoma *in situ*

T1 – tumour invades subepithelial connective tissue

T2 – tumour invades corpus spongiosum, prostate, periurethral muscle

T3 – tumour invades corpus cavernosum, anterior vagina, bladder neck

T4 – tumour invades other adjacent organs

**N – Regional lymph nodes**

NX – regional nodes cannot be assessed

N0 – no regional node metastasis

N1 – metastasis in single lymph node (< 2 cm in diameter)

N2 – metastasis in single lymph node (> 2 cm in diameter), or multiple lymph nodes

**M – Distant metastases**

MX – metastasis cannot be assessed

M0 – no metastasis

M1 – evidence of distant spread

# BIBLIOGRAPHY

## THE NORMAL BLADDER

Caldamone AA. Clinical embryology of the urinary tract. In Weiss RM, George NJR, O'Reilly PH, eds. Comprehensive Urology, 1st edn. London: Mosby International, 2001: 15–30

De Groat WC. Anatomy and physiology of the lower urinary tract. Urol Clin North Am 1993; 20: 383–401

George NJR. Bladder and urethra: function and dysfunction. In Weiss RM, George NJR, O'Reilly PH, eds. Comprehensive Urology, 1st edn. London: Mosby International, 2001: 67–80

Gosling JA, Dixon JS. Applied anatomy of the urinary tract. In Weiss RM, George NJR, O'Reilly PH, eds. Comprehensive Urology, 1st edn. London: Mosby International, 2001: 31–46

Hayes WS. The urinary bladder. In Davidson AS, Hartman DS, eds. Radiology of the Kidney and Urinary Tract. Philadelphia: WB Saunders, 1994: 607–10

McNeal JE. Regional morphology and pathology of the prostate. Am J Clin Pathol 1968; 49: 347–57

McNeal JE. The zonal anatomy of the prostate. Prostate 1981; 2: 35–49

Patel U, Rickards D. Handbook of Transrectal Ultrasound and Biopsy of the Prostate. London: Martin Dunitz, 2002

Waugh A, Grant A. Ross and Wilson Anatomy and Physiology in Health and Illness, 9th edn. London: Churchill Livingstone, 2001: 349–51

## IMAGING MODALITIES USED FOR ASSESSMENT OF THE BLADDER

Baker S, Middleton WD. Color Doppler sonography of ureteral jets in normal volunteers: importance of relative specific gravity in the urine and bladder. Am J Roentgenol 1992; 159: 773–5

Chapple CR, MacDiarmid S. Urodynamics Made Easy, 2nd edn. Edinburgh: Churchill Livingstone, 2000

Grainger RG, Allison DJ, Adam A, Dixon AK, eds. Grainger and Allison's Diagnostic Radiology. A Textbook of Medical Imaging, Vol. 2, 4th edn. London: Churchill Livingstone, 2001

Mundy AR, Stephenson TP, Wein AJ, eds. Urodynamics – Principles, Practice and Application, 2nd edn. Edinburgh: Churchill Livingstone, 1994

Patel U, Kellett MJ. Ureteric drainage and peristalsis post-stenting. Br J Urol 1996; 77: 530–5

Price CL, Adler ES, Rubin JM. Ultrasound detection of differences in density: explanation of ureteric jet phenomenon and implications for new ultrasound applications. Invest Radiol 1989; 24: 876–83

## CONGENITAL ANOMALIES OF THE BLADDER

Bouvier JF, Pascaud E, Maihes F, et al. Urachal cysts in the adult: ultrasonic diagnosis. J Clin Ultrasound 1984; 12: 48

Dunetz GN, Bauer SB. Complete duplication of the bladder and urethra. Urology 1985; 15: 179–84

Friedland GW, Devries PA, Nino-Murcia M, et al. Congenital anomalies of the urinary tract. In Pollack HM, ed. Clinical Urography: An Atlas and Textbook of Urologic Imaging. Philadelphia: WB Saunders, 1990: 559–787

Richman TS, Taylor KJW. Sonographic demonstration of bladder duplication. Am J Roentgenol 1982; 139: 604

Spataro RF, Davis RS, McLachlan MSF, et al. Urachal abnormalities in the adult. Radiology 1983; 149: 659–63

Schiff M Jr, Lytton B. Congenital diverticulum of the bladder. J Urol 1970; 104: 111

Whiter P, Lebowitz RL. Exstrophy of the bladder. Radiol Clin North Am 1977; 15: 93

Yu JS, Kim KW, Lee HJ, et al. Urachal remnant diseases: spectrum of CT and US findings. Radiographics 2001; 21: 451–61

## INTRALUMINAL ABNORMALITIES OF THE BLADDER

Amendola MA, Sonda LP, Diokno AC, Vidyasagar M. Bladder calculi complicating intermittent clean catheterisation. Am J Roentgenol 1983; 141: 751

Chelfouh N, Grenier N, Higueret D, et al. Characterization of urinary calculi: in vitro study of 'twinkling artifact' revealed by color-flow sonography. Am J Roentgenol 1998; 171: 1055–60

Lam AH, Tang S. Sonographic findings in bladder haematoma. Austr Radiol 1194; 38: 48–50

Rifkin MD, Needleman L, Kurtz AB, et al. Sonography of non-gynaecologic cystic masses of the pelvis. Am J Roentgenol 1984; 142: 1169

Rosenfield AT, Taylor KJW, Weiss RM. Ultrasound evaluation of bladder calculi. J Urol 1979; 121: 119

## ABNORMALITIES OF THE BLADDER WALL OR MURAL ABNORMALITIES

Abu Yousef MM, Narayana AS, Brown RC, et al. Urinary bladder tumours studied by cystosonography I. Detection. Radiology 1984; 149: 563

Al-Shorab MM. Radiological manifestations of genito-urinary bilharziasis. Clin Radiol 1968; 19: 100

Brun B, Gammelgaard J, Christoffersen J. Transabdominal dynamic ultrasonography in the detection of bladder tumours. J Urol 1984; 132: 19–20

Buchanan WM, Gelfand M. Calcification of the bladder in urinary schistosomiasis. Trans R Soc Trop Med Hyg 1970; 64: 593–6

Cartoni C, Arcese W, Avvisati G, et al. Role of ultrasonography and follow-up of haemorrhagic cystitis after bone marrow transplantation. Bone Marrow Transplant 1993; 12: 463–7

Corrigna NT, Crooks J, Shand J. Are dedicated bladder films necessary as part of intravenous urography for haematuria. BJU Int 2000; 85: 806–10

Curran FT. Malakoplakia of the bladder. Br J Urol 1987; 59: 559

Das KM, Indudhara R, Vaidyanathan S. Sonographic features of genitourinary tuberculosis. Am J Roentgenol 1992; 158: 327–9

Datta SN, Allen GM, Evans R, et al. Urinary tract ultrasonography in the evaluation of haematuria – a report of 1000 cases. Ann R Coll Surg Engl 2002; 84: 203–5

Doehring E, Ehrich JH, Bremer HJ. Reversibility of urinary tract abnormalities due to *Schistosoma haematobium* infection. Kidney Int 1986; 30: 582–5

Itzcha KY, Singer D, Fischelovitch Y. Ultrasonographic detection of bladder tumours 1. Tumour detection. J Urol 1981; 126: 31

Kauzlauric D, Barmeir E. Sonography of emphysematous cystitis. J Ultrasound Med 1985; 4: 319–20

Khadra MH, Pickard RS, Charlton M, et al. A prospective evaluation of 1930 patients with haematuria to evaluate current diagnostic practice. J Urol 2000; 163: 524–7

Kumar R, Haque AK, Cohen MS. Endometriosis of the urinary bladder demonstrated by sonography. J Clin Ultrasound 1984; 12: 363

Malone PR, Weston-Underwood J, Aron PM, et al. The use of abdominal ultrasound in the detection of early bladder tumours. Br J Urol 1986; 58: 520–2

Pakter R, Nussbaum A, Fishman EK. Haemangioma of the bladder: sonographic and computerized tomography findings. J Urol 1988; 140: 601–2

Pollack HM, Bauner MP, Martinez LO, Hodson CJ. Diagnostic considerations in urinary bladder wall calcification. Am J Roentgenol 1981; 136: 791

Premkumar A, Lattimer J, Newhouse JH. CT and sonography of advanced urinary tract tuberculosis. Am J Roentgenol 1987; 148: 65–9

Raja G, Anson KA, Patel U. Cystitis cystica and cystitis glandularis – presentation with acute ureteric obstruction. Clin Radiol Extra 2003; 58: 43–4

RCR working party. Making the Best Use of a Department of Clinical Radiology, 5th edn. London: The Royal College of Radiologists, 2003

Spencer J, Lindsell D, Mastorakou I. Ultrasonography compared with intravenous urography in the investigation of adults with haematuria. Br Med J 1990; 301: 1396–7

Stark GL, Feddersen R, Lowe BA, et al. Inflammatory pseudotumor (pseudosarcoma) of the bladder. J Urol 1989; 141: 610–12

Steele B, Vade A, Lim-Dunham J. Sonographic appearance of bladder malakoplakia. Pediatr Radiol 2003; 33: 253–5

Vallencien G, Veillon B, Charton M, Brisste JM. Can transabdominal ultrasonography of the bladder replace cystoscopy in the follow-up of superficial bladder tumours. J Urol 1986; 136: 32–4

Zerin JM, Smith JD, Sanvordenker JK, Bloom DA. Sonography of the bladder after ureteral reimplantation. J Ultrasound Med 1992; 11: 87–91

## STAGING OF BLADDER CANCER

Barents JO, Jaeger GJ, van Iverson PB, et al. Staging urinary bladder cancer after transurethral biopsy: value of fast dynamic contrast-enhanced MR imaging. Radiology 1996; 201: 185–93

Devonec M, Chapelon JY, Codas H, et al. Evaluation of bladder cancer with a miniature high frequency transurethral ultrasonographic probe. Br J Radiol 1987; 59: 550–3

Husband J. Bladder cancer. In Husband J, Resnick R, eds. Imaging in Oncology, 1st edn. Oxford: Isis Medical Media, 1998

Kim B, Semelka RC, Ascher SM, et al. Bladder tumor staging: comparison of contrast-enhanced CT, T1- and T2-weighted MR imaging, dynamic gadolinium-enhanced imaging, and late gadolinium-enhanced imaging. Radiology 1994; 193: 239–45

Kim JK, Park SY, Ahn HJ, et al. Bladder cancer: analysis of multi-detector row helical CT enhancement pattern and accuracy in tumor detection and perivesical staging. Radiology 2004; 231: 725–31

Singer D, Itzchak Y, Fishelovitch Y. Ultrasonographic assessment of bladder tumours. 11. Clinical staging. J Urol 1981; 126: 34–6

## ABNORMAL BLADDER CONTOUR OR SIZE

Grainger RG, Allison DJ, Adam A, Dixon AK, eds. Grainger and Allison's Diagnostic Radiology. A Textbook of Medical Imaging, Vol. 2, 4th edn. London: Churchill Livingstone, 2001

Jafri SZH, Diokno AC, Amendola MA, eds. Lower Genitourinary Radiology, 1st edn. New York: Springer, 1996

Patel U, Rickards D. Handbook of Transrectal Ultrasound and Biopsy of the Prostate. London: Martin Dunitz, 2002

## FUNCTIONAL ABNORMALITIES OF THE BLADDER

Abrams P. Urodynamics, 2nd edn. London: Springer-Verlag, 1997

Abrams P, Cardozo L, Fall M, et al. The standardization of terminology of lower urinary tract. Neurourol Urodyn 2002; 21: 167–78

Chapple CR, MacDiarmid S. Urodynamics Made Easy, 2nd edn. Edinburgh: Churchill Livingstone, 2000

Mundy AR, Stephenson TP, Wein AJ, eds. Urodynamics – Principles, Practice and Application, 2nd edn. Edinburgh: Churchill Livingstone, 1994

O'Flynn KJ. The neuropathic bladder. In Weiss RM, George NJR, O'Reilly PH, eds. Comprehensive Urology, 1st edn. London: Mosby International, 2001: 509–20

Saxton HM. Urodynamics: the appropriate modality for the investigation of frequency, urgency, incontinence and voiding difficulties. Radiology 1990; 175: 307–16

Schafr W, Abrams P, Liao L, et al. Good urodynamic practices: uroflowmetry, filling cystometry and pressure-flow studies. Neurourol Urodyn 2002; 21: 261–74

## THE NORMAL URETHRA

Bearcroft PWP, Berman LH. Sonography in the evaluation of the male anterior urethra. Clin Radiol 1994; 49: 621–6

Caldamone AA. Clinical embryology of the urinary tract. In Weiss RM, George NJR, O'Reilly PH, eds. Comprehensive Urology, 1st edn. London: Mosby International, 2001; 15–30

De Groat WC. Anatomy and physiology of the lower urinary tract. Urol Clin North Am 1993; 20: 383–401

Gosling JA, Dixon JS. Applied anatomy of the urinary tract. In Weiss RM, George NJR, O'Reilly PH, eds. Comprehensive Urology, 1st edn. London: Mosby International, 2001; 31–46

McAnich JW, Laing FC, Jeffrey RB. Sonourethrography in the evaluation of urethral strictures: a preliminary report. J Urol 1988; 139: 294–7

McCallum RW. The adult male urethra: normal anatomy, pathology and method of urethrography. Radiol Clin North Am 1979; 17: 227

Neitlich JD, Foster HE, Glickman MG, Smith RC. Detection of urethral diverticula in women: comparison of a high resolution spin echo technique with double balloon urethrography. J Urol 1998; 159: 408–10

Patel U, Lees WR. Penile sonography. In Solbiati L, Rizzatto G, eds. Ultrasound of Superficial Structures. London: Churchill Livingstone, 1995

Ryu JA, Kim B. MR Imaging of the male and female urethra. Radiographics 2001; 21: 1169–85

## CONGENITAL ANOMALIES OF THE URETHRA

Appel RA, Kaplan GW, Broc WA, Streit D. Megalourethra. J Urol 1986; 135: 747

Effman El, Lebowitz RL, Colodny AH. Duplication of the urethra. Radiology 1976; 119: 179

Gonzales ET. Posterior urethral valves and other urethral anomalies. In Walsh PC, Retik AB, Stamey TA, Vaughan ED, eds. Campbell's Urology, 6th edn. Philadelphia: WB Saunders, 1992: 1872–92

Kirks DR, Grossman H. Congenital saccular anterior urethral diverticulum. Radiology 1981; 140: 367

Macpherson RI, Leithiser RE, Gordon L, Turner WR. Posterior urethral valves: an update and review. Radiographics 1986; 6: 753

Merchant SA, Amonkar PP, Patil JA. Imperforate syringocoeles of the bulbourethral duct: appearance on urethrography, sonography and CT. Am J Roentgenol 1997; 169: 823–4

## INTRALUMINAL ABNORMALITIES AND FILLING DEFECTS OF THE URETHRA

Kimche D, Lask D. Congenital polyp of the prostatic urethra. J Urol 1982; 127: 134

McCallum RW. The adult male urethra: normal anatomy, pathology and method of urethrography. Radiol Clin North Am 1979; 17: 227

## INTRINSIC ABNORMALITIES OF THE URETHRAL WALL

El-Mekresh M. Urethral pathology. Curr Opin Urol 2000; 10: 381–90

Harrison WO. Gonoccocal urethritis. Urol Clin North Am 1984; 11: 45

McCallum RW. The adult male urethra: normal anatomy, pathology and method of urethrography. Radiol Clin North Am 1979; 17: 227

Pavlica P, Menchi I, Barozzi L. New imaging of the male anterior urethra. Abdom Imaging 2003; 28: 180–6

Zinman L. Urethral stricture disease. In Weiss RM, George NJR, O'Reilly PH, eds. Comprehensive Urology, 1st edn. London: Mosby International, 2001: 565–82

## LOWER URINARY TRACT TRAUMA

Ali M, Safriel Y, Sciafani SJA, Schulze R. CT signs of urethral injury. Radiographics 2002; 23: 951

Chapple CR. Urethral injury. BJU Int 2000; 86: 318–26

Goldman SM, Sandler CM, Corriere JN, McGuire EJ. Blunt urethral trauma a unified, anatomical mechanical classification. J Urol 1997; 157: 85–9

Gomez RG, Ceballos L, Coburn M, et al. Consensus statement on bladder injuries. BJU Int 2004; 94: 27–32

Hartanto VH, Nitti VW. Recent advances in the management of female lower urinary tract trauma. Curr Opin Urol 2003; 13: 279–84

Vaccoro JP, Brody JM. CT cystography in the evaluation of major bladder trauma. Radiographics 2000; 20: 1373–81

## NEOPLASMS OF THE URETHRA

Mostofi FK, Davis CJ, Sesterhenn IA. Carcinoma of the male and female urethra. Urol Clin North Am 1992; 19: 257–76

Ryu JA, Kim R. MR imaging of the male and female urethra. Radiographics 2001; 21: 1169–85

Wasserman NF. Urethral neoplasm. In Pollack HM, McClennan BL, eds. Clinical Urography, 2nd edn. Philadelphia: WB Saunders, 2000: 1699–715

# Index

absent/small bladder 25, 57, 68
adenocarcinoma, bladder wall 46–67
air, in bladder 33
anterior urethral diverticulum (and megalourethra) 99
ascending urethrography, male 89–91
augmented bladder 61, 63–4

bladder, abnormal shape/size 59–6
   displaced 60–1
   large volume 58
   pear-shaped 59–60
   postoperative appearances 61–4
   small volume 57
bladder calculi 11, 29–31
bladder cancer 43–7, 49–56
   adenocarcinoma 46–7
   incidence 50
   paraganglioma 46
   rhabdomyosarcoma 47
   risk factors 49
   squamous cell carcinoma 46
   staging 49–56
      computed tomography (CT) 14, 53–6
      magnetic resonance imaging (MRI) 53–6
      TNM classification 51
      ultrasound 51–3
   transitional cell carcinoma 43–6
bladder, congenital anomalies 25–8
   absent or small bladder 25
   diverticula 25–7, 35
   duplication anomalies 25
   exstrophy 25
   prune belly syndrome 27
   urachal abnormalities 27–8

bladder filling, terminology of measurements 17
bladder, functional abnormalities 65–86
    abnormal emptying 67, 76–80
        bladder outflow obstruction (BOO) 67, 73, 76–9
        detrusor weakness 67, 80
        poor sphincter relaxation (or dyssynergia) 67, 78–80
    abnormal storage 67, 68–76
        incontinence and sphincter incompetence 67, 72–6
        overactivity (unstable bladder or detrusor overactivity) 67, 68–72
        reduced functional capacity 68
        small volume bladder 68
    neuropathic bladder 82–6
    post-prostate surgery dysfunction 80–2
bladder haemorrhage 31–2
bladder imaging 7–24
    computed tomography (CT) 14, 53–6
    cystography 8–10
    intravenous urogram 8
    magnetic resonance imaging (MRI) 15–16, 53–6
    plain abdominal radiograph 7–8
    ultrasound 10–13, 51–3
        normal bladder 11–13
    *see also* videourodynamics
bladder infections 37–40
    acute cystitis 37–9
    chronic inflammation 40
    emphysematous cystitis 33–4
    haemorrhagic cystitis 39
    infiltration 40
    schistosomiasis 39
    tuberculosis 39
bladder, intraluminal abnormalities 29–34
    blood clot 31–2
    foreign bodies 34
    gas 32–4
    haemorrhage 31–2
    stones 29–31
bladder, normal 1–6
    anatomy 1–4
    embryology 1
    micturition control 5–6, 66–8

neural control of storage/expulsion 5–6

relations 3

shape and size 57

bladder outflow obstruction (BOO) 67, 73, 76–9

causes 76

bladder sensation 17

bladder trauma 115–16

bladder wall abnormalities 35–7

calcification 36–7, 34

cystitis cystica 40

rare anomalies 42

thickening 35–6, 43

tumours 42–7

see also bladder cancer

blood clot, bladder 9, 31–2

Brunn's nests, cystitis cystica 40

Buck fascia 118

calcification, bladder wall abnormalities 9, 37, 34

calculi

bladder 11, 29–31

urethra 103–4

computed tomography (CT) 14

bladder cancer, staging 53–6

contrast urethrography

female 91–2

male 88–91, 120–1

Cowper's duct, in urethritis 109

Cowper's duct cyst 100–1

cystitis

acute 37–9

chronic 40

emphysematous 33–4, 38

haemorrhagic 39

miscellaneous causes 42

radiation cystitis 41

repeated 26

cystitis cystica 40

cystography 8–10

cystourethrography, micturating 90–2

Denonvilliers' fascia 4
detrusor muscle 5–6
    dyssynergia, urodynamics 67, 78–81
    idiopathic (primary) instability 72
    overactivity 17, 67, 68–73
    weakness, abnormal emptying 80
displaced bladder 60–1
duplication anomalies 25

embryology of urinary tract 1
emphysematous cystitis 33, 38
endometriosis 41
external urethral sphincter 6

fistulae, enterovesical 33
flowmetry
    artefacts 19
    examples
        high 73
        post-prostatectomy 84
        reduced 71, 79, 81, 83
    limitations 20
    simple 18, 69
foreign bodies
    bladder 34
    urethra 104–5

gas, bladder 32–4

haematomata, pelvic trauma 59, 116
haemorrhage, bladder 31–2
hair balls, urethra 104
hypospadias 98–99

inclusion bodies 41
incontinence 72–6
    assessment 75
    causes 74
    sphincter relaxation (dyssynergia) 78–81
    stress, and sphincter incompetence 72–7
    urge 72–6

infections *see* bladder infections
infiltration, bladder infection 40
intravenous urography 8–9

lower urinary tract
    trauma 115–21
    urodynamics assessment 16–24
        normal videourodynamics study 23–4
        simple flowmetry 18
        ultrasound cystodynamography (USCD) 18–21
        urodynamics 20–3
lower urinary tract symptoms (LUTS) 65–6
    correlation with abnormal function 67

magnetic resonance imaging (MRI) 15–16
    bladder cancer, staging 53–6
    urethra 95
malakoplakia 41
meatal stenosis 98–9
median umbilical ligament 1
megalourethra and anterior urethral diverticulum 99
Michaeis–Gutmann bodies 41
micturating cystourethrography
    female 91–2
    male 90–2
micturition
    normal control 5–6
    *see also* incontinence
mural abnormalities *see* bladder wall abnormalities

neuropathic bladder 82–6
    complications 86

optical urethrotomy 110

paraganglioma, bladder wall 46
pear-shaped bladder 59–60
pelvic trauma, haematomata 59, 116
*pis-en-deux* 26
plain abdominal radiograph 7–8
polyps, male urethra 105–6, 123–4

posterior urethral valves 97
pouch of Douglas 2, 3
prostate
    anatomy 2, 4–5
    benign hyperplasia, ultrasound cystodynamography (USCD) 18–21
    surgery
        LUTS 82
        postoperative bladder appearance 80–3
        TURP 61
        urodynamics post 84
prostatic urethra 87–8
prostatic utricle 88

radiation cystitis 41
rectovesical pouch 2, 3
reduced functional bladder capacity 67, 68
rhabdomyosarcoma 47

scaphoid megalourethra 99
schistosomiasis 9
    bladder infection 39
sphincter relaxation (dyssynergia), abnormal emptying 78–81
squamous cell carcinoma
    bladder wall 46
    urethra 124–6
stones
    bladder 29–31
    urethra 103–4
stress incontinence, and sphincter incompetence 72–7
surgery, postoperative appearances 61–4
syringocoele (Cowper's duct cyst) 100–1

TNM classification
    bladder cancer 51
    urethral cancer 126
transitional cell carcinoma
    bladder wall 43–6
    urethra 124–6
trauma
    bladder trauma 115–16
    female urethra 121–2

male urethra 116–21

pelvic trauma causing haematomata 59, 116

trigone 1–2

tuberculosis, bladder 39

tumours

bladder wall 42–7

urethra 123–6

*see also* bladder cancer

ultrasound 3, 10–13

bladder cancer, staging 51–3

normal bladder 11–13

ultrasound cystodynamography (USCD) 18–21

ultrasound urethrography

female 94–5

male 92–4

unstable bladder 67, 72

urachal abnormalities 27–8

urachus 1

ureteric jets 12–13

ureters, reimplanted 61

urethra, congenital anomalies 97–101

congenital meatal or urethral stenosis 98–9

Cowper's duct cyst 101–2

hypospadias 99–100

megalourethra and anterior urethral diverticulum 99

polyps 105–6, 123–4

posterior urethral valves 97

urethral duplication 98

urethra, intraluminal abnormalities and filling defects 103–6

calculi 103–4

foreign bodies 104–5

hair balls 104

polyps of male urethra 105–6, 123–4

urethra, normal anatomy 87–8

female 88

male 87–8

urethra, radiological investigation 88–95

contrast urethrography

female 91–2

male 88–91, 120–1

magnetic resonance imaging 95
ultrasound urethrography
    female 94–5
    male 92–4
urethral calculi 103–4
urethral diverticula 99, 110–13
urethral duplication 98
urethral injury 116–21
    investigation 119–21
urethral neoplasms 123–6
    benign tumours 123–4
    carcinoma 124–6
    TNM classification 126
    urethral carcinoma 124–6
urethral stenosis 98–9
urethral strictures 107–10
urethral trauma
    female 121–2
    male 116–21
        classification 119
        investigation 119–21
urethral wall, intrinsic abnormalities 107–13
    diverticula
        female 110–13
        male 113
    strictures 107–10
urethritis 107
urethrography
    contrast 88–92, 120–1
    ultrasound 92–5
urethroplasty 110
urethrotomy, optical 110
urge incontinence, and sphincter incompetence 72–6
urinary jets 12–13
urinoma 117
urodynamics 20–4
    assessment 18
    examples 24
        bladder outflow obstruction 79
        contracted bladder 71
        detrusor muscle dyssynergia 81

        detrusor overactivity 73
        detrusor weakness 83
        neuropathic bladder 85
        normal values 23
        oversensitivity 69
        post-prostatectomy 84
        reduced compliance 70
        stress incontinence 77
    terminology of measurements 17
urogenital diaphragm 4
urothelium 2

verumontanum 87–8
videourodynamics 20
    normal 23–4
    technique 22
    *see also* urodynamics
voiding, terminology of measurements 17